Coconut Water

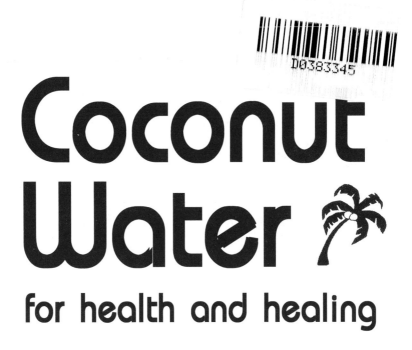

for health and healing

Dr. Bruce Fife

Piccadilly Books, Ltd.
Colorado Springs, CO

Every effort has been made to ensure that the information contained in this book is complete and accurate. However, neither the publisher nor the author is engaged in rendering professional advice or services to the individual reader. The information contained in this book is not intended as a substitute for consulting with your physician. All matters regarding your health require medical supervision. Neither the author nor the publisher shall be liable or responsible for any loss or damage allegedly arising from any information or suggestion in this book.

Copyright © 2008, by Bruce Fife
All rights reserved. No part of this book may be reproduced in any form, except for brief reviews, without written permission from the publisher.

Cover design by Tathy Otero

Piccadilly Books, Ltd.
P.O. Box 25203
Colorado Springs, CO 80936, USA
www.piccadillybooks.com
info@piccadillybooks.com

Library of Congress Cataloging-in-Publication Data

Fife, Bruce, 1952-
    Coconut water for health and healing / by Dr. Bruce Fife.
        p. cm.
    Includes bibliographical references and index.
    ISBN 978-0-941599-66-5
    1. Coconut water--Health aspects. I. Title.
    QP144.C63F54 2007
    613.2'87--dc22
                                                    2007028383

Published in the USA
Printed in Canada
Sold Worldwide

Table of Contents

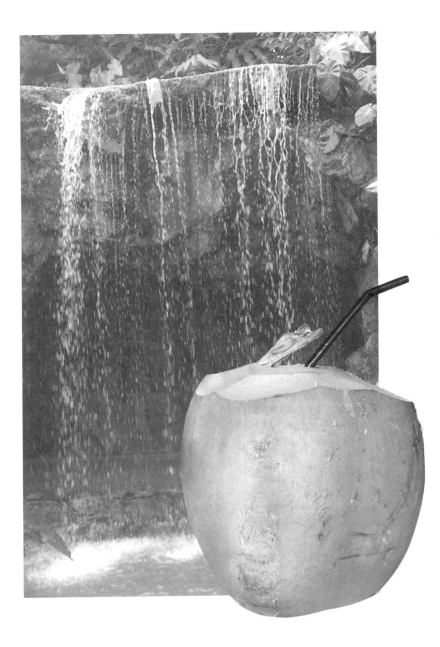

Water of Life

COCONUT WATER SAVED MY LIFE!

The ship's captain couldn't believe his eyes. Off in the distance on the tiny desolate island stood a man dressed only in his underwear and apparently in distress. Desperate to attract the ship's attention, the man vigorously waved a flag made from his clothes and shouted for help.

Weeks earlier a massive earthquake off the coast of Indonesia generated a series of immense tsunamis that devastated thousands of miles of coastline and completely smothered many small islands. The lone survivor, Michael Mangal, was sucked into the sea when the first tsunami wave retreated back into the ocean, but an even bigger second wave dumped him back on shore. However, he found that his village was completely destroyed and no one else had survived. Injured and desperate, he struggled for survival. All food and drinkable water on the island had been ruined, leaving him desolate. The only food available was fallen coconuts that littered the ground and those that still clung tightly to the surviving trees. For the next 25 days Mangal lived solely on coconuts. All drinkable water on the island had been contaminated by seawater and debris. His only source of fluid came from the water inside the coconuts.

When Mangal was rescued, he was in relatively good health despite his harrowing experience and lack of food and water. The coconuts provided him with the nourishment and fluids his body needed to survive. A person can live several weeks without food, but only a few days without water, so procuring a source of drinkable water was essential for Mangal's survival. During his 25 day ordeal the only water available to him was from coconuts. Recalling his experience Mangal said, "Coconut water saved my life!"

In the aftermath of the December 26, 2004 earthquake and the resulting wave of tsunamis, there were many stories similar to Mangal's. People were forced to survive on whatever food was available. Coconuts, which have a hard protective shell, are abundant in the area and were just about the only source of food and water that survived the disaster. Many survival stories appeared in the news. People were swept out to sea and survived by clinging to floating debris, scooping up coconuts floating in the water, and tearing them open with their teeth. Others roamed the countryside for weeks scavenging for food and water, which the coconuts provided. Coconuts literally saved the lives of thousands of people who had their homes and villages destroyed.

The value of coconuts as a source of food and drink is well known among the people on tropical islands around the world. In fact, it is because of the coconut that their ancestors were able to cross thousands of miles of open water. Coconuts were essential because they provided a convenient long-lasting source of nourishment. On many small islands, especially Pacific atolls, the sandy volcanic soil is too porous to hold fresh water. The only source of drinkable water is from the coconut. People have survived for many months, even years with little more to eat and drink than coconut meat and water.

LIVING WATER

The coconut palm is a remarkable plant. It is said to have a thousand uses. Every part of the plant can be used for some purpose. It is used for food, drink, medicine as well as building material for homes, boats, fishing gear, rope, nets, baskets, bowls, floor and bed mats, and clothes, to mention just a few. If you were on a deserted island and the only resource you had available were coconut trees and the knowledge to use them, you could survive. The coconut palm is so vital to the existence of people on the islands that it is called "the tree that provides all things necessary for life" or simply "the tree of life."

6

The coconut is the fruit of the tree of life. Inside the coconut is a most remarkable fluid: coconut water. This is actual "living" water. To say that coconut contains living water is not a figure of speech, it is literal. Coconut water is actually living tissue of the coconut palm.[1] Even months after a coconut has been separated from the tree, it remains alive. Water from a faucet, a stream, a well, or even that purified by the process of reverse osmoses is essentially lifeless. Coconut water, on the other hand, is the fluid or the lifeblood, of a living plant. It is from the coconut water and the meat that a new coconut palm derives its energy and nourishment to sprout and grow into a towering coconut palm.

Coconut water is a superfood filled with minerals, vitamins, amino acids, sugars, enzymes, and growth hormones. It possesses incredible healing properties. It is currently being used around the world to save lives. It is of particular value in the treatment of cholera—a devastating illness in many areas in the world. Cholera is a terrible disease that can strike so fast and with such ferocity that it causes death in as little as 12 hours. Consumption of coconut water increases the survival rate of cholera victims by as much as 97 percent. Coconut water is just as useful in combating influenza, dysentery, salmonella, and E coli. It doesn't necessarily kill the viruses or bacteria that cause the disease, it provides fluids and nutrients that allow the body to successfully fight the battle on its own. It has a normalizing effect and gives the body a boost of power so that it can overcome a number of conditions. It is known to be of benefit in relieving fatigue, constipation, dehydration, kidney and bladder disorders, glaucoma, and cataract. It is reported to turn back time, so to speak, by reversing or slowing down the aging process. It is even reported to increase libido. Coconut is hypoallergenic, meaning those people who have food allergies can usually consume coconut without fear. The water especially is safe because of its low protein content. Coconut water also has an alkalizing effect on the body, helping to counteract or balance the effects of acidifying foods which are so common in our diets.

One of the more remarkable characteristics of coconut water is its chemical profile and mineral content. The primary minerals or electrolytes in coconut water are essentially the same as those found in human blood. For this reason, doctors have used it as an intravenous fluid for rehydration, pumping it directly into the patient's bloodstream. It also makes an ideal oral rehydration beverage. Whether given intravenously or orally, coconut water has saved thousands of lives, mostly children in underdeveloped countries.

Coconut water's similarity to body fluids and its usefulness as an intravenous and oral rehydration fluid has spurred interest in the sports community. With properties which are in many ways superior to commercial sports drinks, coconut water is now becoming popular as a natural rehydration beverage among amateur and professional athletes. Even the non-athletic consumer is discovering the many advantages coconut water has to offer.

YOUNG COCONUTS

The coconut palm is a tropical plant that grows best in hot, humid environments close to the sea. It grows well in sandy soil and brackish water and, therefore, thrives on tropical islands and coastlines around the world. The classical vision of a tropical paradise is lying on the beach under a coconut palm, sipping coconut water through a straw from a fresh young coconut.

It is very important that you understand that *coconut water* is not the same as *coconut milk*. Many people who live outside the tropics and are not accustomed to eating fresh coconuts often confuse these terms. If you've ever held a coconut and shaken it, you will hear liquid sloshing about. This liquid is often mistakenly referred to as coconut "milk." This is not accurate. The liquid inside a coconut is correctly termed "coconut water." Coconut water develops naturally inside the coconut. To get it, all you have to do is open the coconut and pour it out. Coconut milk, on the other hand, is a manufactured product. It is produced by crushing coconut meat and extracting the juice. The two products are completely different in taste, texture, appearance, and nutritional content. Coconut water looks like ordinary water with a slightly cloudy appearance. Sometimes you hear coconut water referred to as coconut juice. Coconut milk, on the other hand, is a solid white color with a creamy texture. It looks just like dairy milk. It is often sold in cans in the grocery store. The focus of this book is on the health aspects of the water.

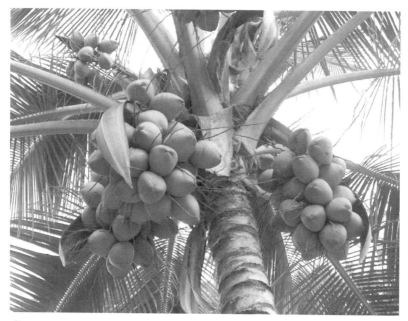

Coconuts at various stages of development.

Coconut palms can grow a hundred feet tall and live for 70 years. Technically, coconuts are classified as drupes—single seeded fruits. Cherries, plums, and olives are also drupes. In the case of the coconut, the flesh surrounding the seed is not edible. This flesh is referred to as the *husk* and is very thick and fibrous. Inside the husk is the seed or kernel. The kernel has a hard shell. Inside the shell wall is a layer of white "meat" and a cavity filled with water. The meat and water are the edible portions of the coconut fruit.

Coconuts grow in bunches usually containing between 5 to 12 fruits. A mature coconut palm normally produces a new bunch every month or about 12 bunches a year. Since the tree is continually producing fruit, coconuts are always in season. A productive coconut palm can yield 100-140 coconuts a year.

Coconuts take between 12-13 months to fully mature. The taste, texture, size, and content of the coconut meat and liquid varies as the fruit matures. A very young coconut, less than 6 months old, is completely filled with liquid and has very little meat. The meat (endosperm) has a

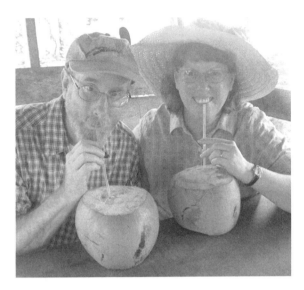

The author and his wife enjoying fresh young coconut water in the Philippines.

soft, jelly-like texture and can be eaten with a spoon. At this stage both the liquid and meat are very sweet and delicious. Coconuts reach full size at about 6-7 months. At this point they are still only halfway developed and will take another 6 months to reach full maturity. As the coconut matures, the amount of liquid decreases and the meat increases in thickness and hardness. At about 10-12 months the liquid to meat ratio is reversed. Fully ripe coconuts have only a small amount of liquid and a thick hard layer of meat. Both the meat and liquid become less sweet with age.

Coconuts contain the greatest amount of liquid at about 8-9 months of age. This is also about the time when they taste the best. In young coconuts most of the sugar is in the form of glucose and fructose. In mature coconuts the sugar content decreases slightly and is predominately sucrose. Protein and fat content also increases with age, but even then the amount is very small. Young coconut water is essentially fat free.

If you travel in the tropics, you may see coconuts of various shapes and sizes. There are many different varieties of coconut: some, with their husk, are as large as a basketball, others as small as baseballs.

The most common type used for food and water are about the size of a bowling ball. The different varieties also have a slightly different flavor. Some are tastier than others, but they are all beneficial.

Mature coconuts, with the husk removed, are the type most commonly found in grocery stores. These are the brown, hairy coconuts with which we are all familiar. In the tropics, however, immature coconuts are among the most popular foods. Immature coconuts are called *young* or *green* coconuts. You may also hear them referred to as *tender* coconuts. The term tender refers to the soft jelly-like meat they contain at this stage of development. The outside husk of a young coconut is usually a dark green color. Some varieties are yellow or orange-red. As the coconut matures, the husk turns brown.

Young coconuts have a thin shell which is relatively easy to crack or puncture. As the coconut matures, the shell hardens. Fully mature shells are very hard and difficult to break open, and frequently require

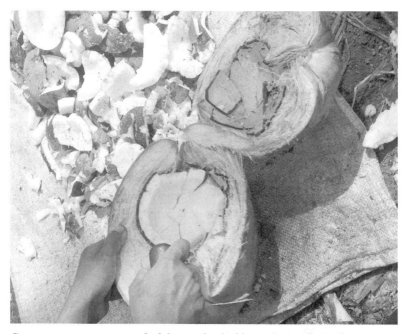

Coconuts are surrounded by a thick fiberous husk. Before going to market the husk is often removed.

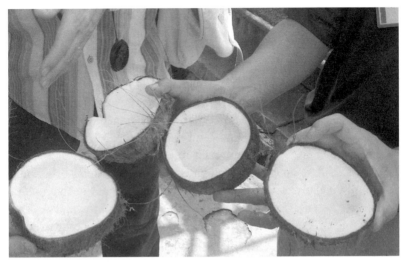

Dehusked mature coconuts. Notice the thick layer of white meat inside the shells. Young coconuts have a very thin layer of meat.

a hammer and a strong set of muscles. Experienced coconut openers can split a coconut in half with just a couple of blows from the dull side of a machete.

A single young coconut typically contains about 12-16 ounces (360-480 ml) of water. Mature coconuts contain considerably less, often no more than 8 ounces (240 ml). Young coconut water makes a refreshing beverage and a super health tonic. Mature coconut water has similar characteristics but is not considered as beneficial nor nearly as tasty, thus it is rarely ever consumed. Contrary to what you might think, coconut water does *not* taste like desiccated coconut. It has a mild, sweet, nutty flavor that doesn't taste at all like the meat you get from a mature coconut.

FOLKLORE AND TRADITION

Coconut has a long history of use throughout the tropical world. Its importance cannot be overstated. Where it grows it is intertwined in the daily life, culture, heritage, cuisine, and commerce of the people.

The coconut makes life possible in many locations, especially where other resources are limited. It is a dependable food source and can be relied on in times of distress or calamities, such as tsunamis or storms that may destroy other sources of food and drink. The sturdy coconut palm can withstand hurricane force winds and harsh conditions that would devastate other plants.

Because of its importance, the coconut plays an central part in the folklore and traditions of the people. It is viewed as a symbol of fertility and prosperity. Its meat and water, as well as the milk and oil which are derived from the meat, are used extensively in foods. In some areas coconut in some form or another is eaten every single day. It has become an integral part of the cuisine of many peoples. Coconut chutney from India, buko pie from the Philippines, vaisalo from Samoa, and Thai curries, are but a few of the traditional dishes using coconut.

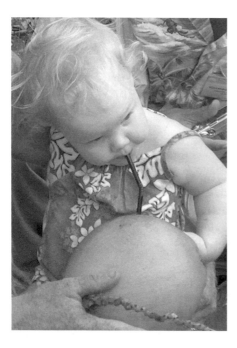

Children love drinking young coconut water.

Coconut water is a popular drink everywhere in the tropics. It is important as a source of liquid and as a health tonic. It is believed to relieve or cure disease and ensure good health. The juice is taken to strengthen the heart and restore energy to those who are ill.

In the islands of the South Pacific all young mothers are encouraged to drink plenty of coconut water to ensure that their breast milk is rich and plentiful and that the baby grows strong and healthy. Often infants are given both mother's milk and coconut water. If a mother can't nurse or if the infant has digestive problems, it is given coconut water. The water and soft meat from immature coconuts are used to wean babies off their mother's milk.

In the Nicobar Islands in the Indian Ocean, coconuts are so highly prized that until the early part of the 20th century they were used as currency to purchase goods.

They are of such value to Samoans that to see one lying on the ground does not mean it is free, but that it must belong to someone who has put it there and will come back for it. If no one is looking and somebody takes the coconut, the tapui, a magical spirit, will punish the thief and bring him misfortune or sickness.

In the Philippines they honor the coconut with an annual Coconut Week celebration. A dozen other countries celebrate September 2 every year as International Coconut Day.

In India the coconut is considered a sacred food and is an essential part of Hindu religious ceremonies and social functions. A dehusked coconut is always a part of temple offerings in southern India where coconuts are plentiful. The coconut is broken and pieces distributed to the congregation as an offering. Coconut is included in weddings as part of the ceremony. It is used to ward off misfortune and symbolizes selfless service of the wedding couple to each other. The food served to wedding guests always includes coconut in some form. When a building project is inaugurated, be it religious or civil, a coconut is smashed on the ground or on some object as part of an initiation process; this act signifies a sacrifice of ego, the idea that wealth stems from divinity, and the belief that, if due credit is not given, bad karma will result.

Coconuts have been used in India for thousands of years. They are prized for their nutritional and health benefits. The juice from young coconuts is regarded as the most nutritious and wholesome beverage that nature has provided for the people. It is considered to be an effective aphrodisiac, diuretic, detoxifier, liver rejuvenator, and all-around health tonic. Taken orally it is used as an anti-intoxication agent to relieve drunkenness. Whenever someone is sick, coconut water is usually part of the treatment to nourish the patient back to health. According to tradition, young coconut water is useful in treating the following conditions:

Cancer
Constipation
Dehydration
Diabetes
Diarrhea
Fatigue
Heat boils
Hives
Heatstroke
Intestinal worms
Intoxication
Itching
Jaundice
Kidney stones
Male sterility
Measles
Nausea
Nervousness
Osteoporosis
Pimples
Prickly heat (heat rash)
Sunburn
Urinary tract infections

When rubbed on the skin, coconut water can reduce rashes, including those caused by hives, small pox, chicken pox, and measles. Mixed with rice flour, it makes a healing poultice for gangrenous ulcers, skin boils, and other infections. When the water is applied to the face, it is believed to remove wrinkles.

Throughout the course of history, coconut water has proven itself an effective healer and rejuvenator. Whether it can do all the things it is purported to do is yet to be proven. However, modern medical research is demonstrating the truth of many of the claims. In the following chapters you will discover what medical science has learned up to this point. Quite honestly, the benefits are nothing short of astounding. Further research is bound to confirm more of the historical uses and perhaps discover new uses for the water in treating disease and restoring health.

2

Intravenous Use of Coconut Water

THE MIRACLE WATER THAT SAVES LIVES

In one of Jackie Chan's movies, he plays a character who is seriously injured and left to die in a remote tropical area. Struggling to survive, he begins treating himself with the resources available. Coconut palms were growing nearby. Taking a fresh coconut, he inserts a hollow reed though one of the "eyes" and inserts the other end of the reed into a vein in his arm. The liquid from the coconut drains into his bloodstream, bringing about a quick recovery.

While this story is fictional, the use of coconut water as an intravenous (IV) fluid is not. Intravenous therapy is the process of delivering fluids and nutrients directly into the bloodstream by way of a vein. When oral delivery is too slow or not possible, IV therapy becomes necessary. Coconut water IV therapy has been around for over 60 years. When commercial IV solution has not been available, coconut water has successfully taken its place.

During World War II it is reported that British doctors used intravenous coconut water in Ceylon as did the Japanese in Sumatra and doctors under American jurisdiction in the Caroline Islands in the South Pacific. Dr. Arobati Hicking, a Micronesian working in the Caroline Islands during the war, reported successfully using coconut water injections on at least 20 patients suffering from dehydration and severe malnutrition.[1] While working in Uganda in the early 1960s, Dr. D. B. Jelliffe used coconut water infusions to successfully treat patients

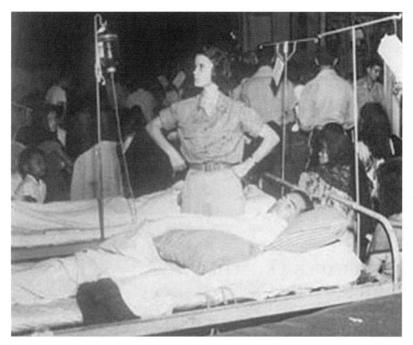

Nurse administering intravenous therapy to wounded soldier during World War II.

suffering from starvation and nutritional edema.[2] Later coconut water was used again in military field hospitals during the Vietnam War and during the Nigerian Civil War of 1967-1970. Dr. E. O. Olurin recalls that during the Nigerian conflict they were compelled to administer coconut water intravenously for the resuscitation of wounded soldiers as a result of a temporary shortage of medical supplies. At the time the doctors weren't aware of any previous work on the intravenous use of coconut water. They used coconut water because they had nothing else at their disposal. Their results on the battlefield were so encouraging that by the end of the war, they began a formal study of this use of coconut water.[3] Over the years coconut water has been used successfully as an intravenous fluid on numerous occasions.

In remote regions of the world, medical resources used for intravenous hydration and resuscitation of critically ill patients are limited. When faced with shortages, physicians have to improvise with the available resources or do without. An incident reported in the *American Journal of Emergency Medicine* in 2000 at the Atoifi hospital in the South Pacific provides an excellent example.

Atoifi hospital is a 100-bed facility on the island of Malaita in the Solomon Islands. The village of Atoifi is nestled in the jungle on the east side of the island. The only way to get there is by small fixed-wing airplane or boat. Two other hospitals serve Malaita, but travel between them is difficult because of the mountainous jungle topography and the absence of roads.

On November 23, 1999 an adult male in his forties was admitted to the hospital. While at home, he collapsed to the floor for no apparent reason. He had experienced four similar episodes on previous occasions but had not sought medical treatment. He had lost control of the left side of his body from his feet to his head. That side of his face drooped and saliva pooled in his mouth. He had suffered a stroke.

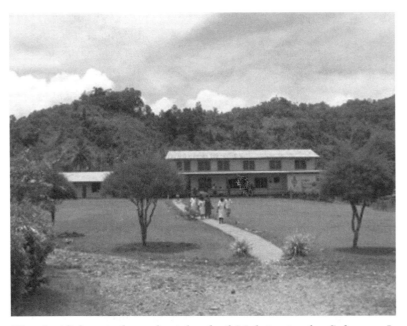

The Atoifi hospital on the island of Malaita in the Solomon Islands.

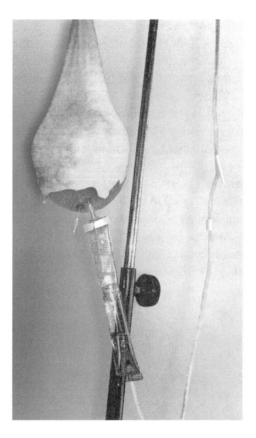

Intravenous coconut water set-up. The coconut is suspended above the patient with orthopedic netting. A needle is injected into one of the soft "eyes" of the coconut to equalize pressure. A second needle attached to blood transfusion tubing is inserted into another eye. Coconut water flows through the tubing to a needle which is inserted into the vein of the patient.

The following day he had difficulty swallowing and was temporarily given a standard IV saline solution for rehydration. The patient continued to have difficulty and was choking on both solids and liquids, so tube feeding was initiated. He complained of discomfort from the tube but refused the option of having a tube surgically placed into his stomach.

The patient remained in the hospital for 36 days with no improvement. In fact, his condition got worse. He became weak, shaky, and dizzy. He was unable to tolerate the tube feedings and began vomiting. Intravenous hydration again became necessary.

The hospital's remaining supply of IV solution was quickly exhausted. The nearest hospital was on the other side of the island and would take a full day's travel to reach. In addition, the hospital did not have the financial resources to fly supplies in from the capital city of Honiara, which was on another island a hundred miles away.

The physicians at the hospital had heard that coconut water had been used successfully in emergency situations on other islands. With the patient on death's doorstep and no other options available, the doctors decided to take this approach. Immature coconuts were gathered and dehusked. A needle was inserted into the soft eye of the coconut. Blood transfusion tubing connected this needle to a vein in the patient's arm, allowing the coconut water to be delivered directly into his bloodstream.

The patient received coconut water in this manner for the next two days. During this time his health made a dramatic turn for the better. He regained the ability to swallow and progressed so rapidly that he was released from the hospital the following day.[4]

What a remarkable story! The patient suffered for 36 days in the hospital. His condition grew worse each day, even with the aid of commercial IV solution. When he was given coconut water, his health abruptly returned and after just two days he was well enough to be released from the hospital and go home. This miracle water literally saved his life. What is in the fluid of a fresh (living) coconut that can restore health and bring someone back from the brink of death? Whatever it is, it is apparently not found in commercial IV solution which had little effect on this patient.

ALMOST LIKE HUMAN BLOOD PLASMA

Using the juice from the inside of a coconut as an IV solution is not as bizarre as it might sound. The composition of coconut water is remarkably similar to human blood plasma. Like human blood plasma it contains a mixture of sugars, minerals, amino acids, vitamins, hormones, and other substances necessary for growth and development. It is the lifeblood of the plant embryo.

For IV use the most suitable water comes from an immature coconut about 7-9 months old. If the coconut is fresh (i.e., still living) and undamaged, the water inside is completely free from harmful bacteria or fungus and can be injected directly into the bloodstream without further sterilization. In fact, studies show that heat sterilized coconut water is less suitable for IV use and increases the risk of irritation at the insertion point.

Immature or young coconut water has only trace amounts of fat and very little protein. The absence of protein is an advantage because proteins give the most trouble by causing immune reactions. Although there is not much protein, the water does contain many essential amino acids including lysine, leucine, cysteine, phenylalanine, histidine, and tryptophan. The major minerals in coconut water are the same as those in human blood plasma. These minerals are sodium, potassium, chloride, calcium, phosphorus, magnesium, and sulfur, with trace amounts of many others. The minerals are in the form of ions, which are electrically charged atoms and molecules. These charged mineral ions are referred to as *electrolytes*. The major difference in the mineral or electrolyte content in blood and coconut water is that plasma contains a higher percentage of sodium and coconut water contains a higher percentage of potassium. But the major electrolytes are essentially the same. The sugars present are primarily in the form of glucose and fructose. This combination of nutrients makes coconut water exceptionally well suited for IV use.

CLINICAL RESEARCH

Clinical experience has shown that coconut water is accepted favorably by the body without stimulating an immune response or causing unwanted reactions. The only thing that keeps it from being an ideal IV fluid is its relatively low sodium content compared to human blood plasma. This apparent shortcoming is easily solved simply by adding a little salt (sodium chloride) to the water. However, even without the added salt, coconut water has proven its worth as an acceptable IV solution.

The basic chemical composition of coconut water has been known at least since the 1930s. Its similarity to human blood plasma was apparently noticed by doctors who reasoned that it might make a suitable intravenous solution. Experiments with animals in the early 1940s proved so successful that human trials were soon initiated. The first clinical study using human subjects reported in the medical literature was published in 1942.[5] In this study 12 hospitalized children were given coconut water IVs as part of their treatment. The children tolerated the coconut water well without any adverse effects, demonstrating that coconut water can be used as an IV solution in humans. Perhaps because of this study, Japanese and British military doctors turned to IV coconut water during the Second World War.[6]

The effectiveness of intravenous use of coconut water was proven on the battlefield. After the war, a number of studies on coconut water as an emergency replacement for standard IV solution were published in medical journals around the world.[7-21] Researchers from Britain, New Zealand, India, Thailand, Indonesia, Africa, the Philippines, Malaysia, and even the United States performed studies on the use of coconut water as an intravenous fluid in human subjects. In all cases, the subjects tolerated the coconut well, without any serious adverse effects.

The consensus among the studies is that fresh coconut water is a suitable substitute for commercial IV solutions. What makes coconut water useful is that it is naturally sterile (i.e., free of germs), has a chemical profile similar to—although not quite identical to—blood plasma, is readily available in many parts of the world, is inexpensive and easy to use, is low in protein and does not cause immune or allergic reactions, is well tolerated by the body, supplies essential nutrients, causes no harm, and supplies much needed fluid.

Other constituents of the water such as plant hormones, enzymes, and antioxidants may exert unknown health benefits. Although coconut water is not completely identical to blood plasma or commercial IV solution, it appears to be equally as effective and perhaps even superior in some ways, as evidenced in the patient at the Atoifi hospital who recovered in less than two days with the use of coconut water.

In a more recent study by German scientists, coconut water was tested for its ability to scavenge free radicals that interfere with the function of hemoglobin.[22] Hemoglobin is the molecule in red blood cells that carries and delivers oxygen throughout our bodies. The researchers found that fresh coconut water was effective in neutralizing free radicals and protecting hemoglobin from nitrite-induced oxidation. Oxidation of hemoglobin is a destructive action which hampers the body's ability to effectively transport oxygen and remove carbon dioxide. The maturity of the coconut was important. Young or immature coconut water displayed the greatest antioxidant protection. As the coconut matures, this protective effect decreases. Fresh coconut water was more effective than acid, alkali, or heat-treated coconut water. Apparently the water works best just as nature makes it.

In animal and human studies, as well as in numerous emergency situations in times of war and peace, coconut water has proven to be safe and useful. Harry Goldsmith, MD in his review of IV coconut water therapy published in 1962 states, "all recorded instances of intravenous coconut water being used, no serious reactions have *ever* been noted [emphases mine].[23] This observation is repeated in a more

MAJOR ELECTROLYTES IN BODY FLUIDS AND COCONUT WATER

Electrolyte	Extracellular Fluid (mEq/L)	Intracellular Fluid (mEq/L)	Coconut Water (mEq/L)
Sodium (Na^+)	142	10	5
Potassium (K^+)	5	150	49
Calcium (Ca^{++})	5	2	12
Magnesium (Mg^{++})	3	40	17
Chloride (Cl^-)	103	2	63
Phosphate $(HPO_4^=)$	2	103	8
Sulfate $(SO_4^=)$	1	20	5

The major electrolytes in coconut water are exactly the same as those found in extracellular and intracellular fluids. However the quantity of each electrolyte in coconut water does not match exactly with either the extracellular or intracellular fluids. Instead it is more like a mixture of the two. Since dehydration affects both extracellular and intracellular fluids, electrolytes from both compartments need to be replaced, which coconut water does quite well.

Coconut water values from Eiseman, B. Intravenous infusion of coconut water. *A.M.A. Archives of Surgerey* 1954;68:167-178.

recent statement by Darilyn Campbell-Falck, MD and colleagues in 2000. After an extensive review of published studies and case reports stated, "there have been no adverse affects reported."[24]

ANSWERING THE SKEPTICS
I have written briefly about the intravenous use of coconut water in a previous book.[25] After reading this book a reader approached her doctor and asked him if it was possible. His response was classic, "Why of course not. That's ridiculous!" The patient felt embarrassed and humiliated for even asking. Like most doctors, he had not studied the issue and was completely unfamiliar with the studies. Because of his prejudice and lack of knowledge on the subject, he rejected the idea and flatly rebuked the patient. On the whole, doctors are skeptical of any treatment that isn't a product of the pharmaceutical industry. Despite its record of safety, the use of coconut water as an intravenous solution is no exception. Most doctors seem to have a hard time accepting the fact that coconut water can be as good as commercial IV solutions.

While researchers will admit coconut water is suitable as a replacement for commercial IV solution, some caution that it should only be used for a limited time and only in emergency situations. Some physicians express caution because putting something like coconut water into a person's vein just doesn't seem right to them regardless of its proven track record. It is hard for these people to believe that something from nature can be as good as, or even better than, the products of modern chemistry. To justify their position critics note a few possible areas of concern.

One of the points they bring out is that young coconut water is more acidic (pH 4.2-5.4) than plasma (pH 7.4). Some researchers have expressed concern that injecting coconut water into the bloodstream may upset the blood's acid-alkaline balance. However, studies show that blood pH is not adversely affected by the coconut water.[26] Blood pH remains normal. The overall effect seems to be more alkalizing because patient's urine becomes noticeably more alkaline. The reason why is probably due to its high concentration of potassium, calcium, and magnesium, all of which have an alkalizing effect in the body. A similar situation occurs when eating lemons, which are acidic, but have an alkalizing effect on the body. Like lemons, the acidity of coconut water is caused by the presence of small amounts of citric acid and ascorbic acid (vitamin C). When the pH of coconut water is altered purposely to make it more alkaline, it decreases the water's effectiveness and increases the risk of adverse reactions. So the slight acidity appears not to have any detrimental effect.

Although the major minerals in coconut water are the same as those in plasma, the concentrations are somewhat different. Coconut water has a higher concentration of potassium and magnesium. Some researchers have expressed concern that a large amount of coconut water given intravenously might upset mineral balance. They point out that commercial solutions containing a large amount of these electrolytes can disrupt a patient's mineral balance and so patients must be carefully monitored. However, this doesn't seem to be the case with coconut water. The combination of minerals and other constituents in coconut water apparently allows the body to effectively excrete excess minerals and retain those in which the body is deficient, so a balance is always maintained.[27-28] Even though the water contains a high amount of potassium, patients receiving relatively large quantities of IV coconut water do not show abnormally high potassium levels. Yet patients with sodium deficiencies show marked improvement in sodium levels.[29] Unlike commercial IV solutions which simply pump minerals into the bloodstream and may cause an excess, coconut water seems to have the ability to normalize or balance the body's electrolyte levels.

The biggest concern expressed by some researchers is the relatively low percentage of sodium and high percentage of potassium as compared to plasma. This ratio of sodium to potassium causes concern because it creates a diuretic (increased urine flow) effect that might promote dehydration rather than relieve it. One of the main uses of IV therapy is to replace fluids that have been lost and to reverse dehydration. Giving a patient a solution that causes more fluids to be lost through urine would promote dehydration.

In 1954 Dr. B. Eiseman and colleagues tested this theory on five patients. The patients received intravenous coconut water as their only source of fluid for 24 hours. Total urinary output was measured during this time. The amount of fluid excreted exceeded the amount infused, demonstrating that there was a diuretic effect. Eiseman concluded that

IV coconut water had no clinical value in improving dehydration although he conceded that it could be useful in certain situations: such as to provide potassium or calories, increase blood volume (due to loss of blood), or as a vehicle for the injection of sodium salts.[30]

The fact that IV coconut water has been used very successfully as a rehydration fluid contrasts with Dr. Eiseman's findings. Although several possible reasons would account for this discrepancy, Dr. Eiseman's study had one major problem. Eiseman states that before the infusion with coconut water, all five subjects were well hydrated, had good urinary output, and were not acutely ill. In other words, they were all in fairly good health. This is where the problem lies. Coconut water apparently won't over-hydrate a person who is already adequately hydrated. This is a good thing because too much water can be just as harmful as too little.

Eiseman states that IV coconut water can be useful in the case of hypokalemia—a potentially fatal condition in which blood potassium levels become very low. Hypokalemia can result from a variety of medical conditions. The most common cause is as a result of excessive water loss which carries potassium out of the body. Typically, this is a consequence of vomiting and diarrhea, but may also occur with excessive sweating or from illness or physical exertion. In other words, hypokalemia can occur whenever the patient is *dehydrated!* Since coconut water is rich in potassium, it makes an excellent rehydration fluid. The reason why Eiseman's patients lost excess fluid with the IV coconut water is because they were not dehydrated or potassium deficient. Therefore, the IV coconut water had a diuretic effect on them. In cases were patients have lost a lot of blood or are dehydrated, they need both potassium and fluids, which coconut water can supply. So, contrary to Eiseman's caution, coconut water is ideal for rehydration. This has since been proven in numerous studies using coconut water both intravenously and orally as a treatment for dehydration. Studies have shown that coconut water can be infused by as much as one fourth to one third of the patient's body weight without complications.[31]

The relatively low amount of sodium (as well as chloride) in proportion to potassium is the primary reason for the diuretic effect in coconut water. This effect can be erased, simply by adding ordinary salt (sodium chloride) to the water. The addition of a little salt compensates for this deficiency, making coconut water an excellent replacement for commercial IV solution, even when patients are already properly hydrated.

Commercial IV solution used for rehydration therapy is typically made of sterile water and sodium chloride with or without glucose (sugar). Medications and other substances can also be added. For rehydration the solution is usually just salt and sugar water.

Coconut water's mixture of major minerals, trace minerals, amino acids, vitamins, antioxidants, hormones, enzymes, glucose, fructose, and other substances in many ways more closely resembles blood plasma in its total composition than does commercial solution. Apparently these elements all work together to keep blood chemistry in balance, supply nutrients necessary to facilitate healing, and stimulate recovery. This is witnessed in incidences such as in the Atoifi case where coconut water, even without added salt, was superior to commercial IV solution in rehydrating the patient and stimulating healing.

3

Oral Rehydration

DEHYDRATION NATION

You've had it. I've had it. We've all experienced it to one extent or another sometime in our lives. Many of you right now as you read this are affected by it. What am I talking about? I'm speaking of dehydration.

You don't have to be a competitive athlete or a sports enthusiast to become dehydrated. You don't even have to be physically active. We are all dehydrated to some degree at various times. Often we become so busy at work and in our everyday lives that we don't take the time to satisfy thirst. We put it off until it's more convenient. Ignoring the thirst reflex dulls this sensation. We become so accustomed to ignoring the body's subtle signals of thirst that we don't realize we are becoming dehydrated

If you rely on coffee, tea, or soda for most of your fluids during the day, you are probably chronically dehydrated and don't even realize it. In fact, so many of us are dehydrated that we have become a nation of dehydration.

A study by the National Research Council revealed that on average women (ages 15-49) drink a mere 2.6 cups of water a day. Most of their fluids come from beverages. This finding suggests that a large portion of women may be chronically dehydrated. Another study performed by researchers at Johns Hopkins Hospital in Baltimore discovered that 32-41 percent of the subjects they tested (both men and women ages 23-44) were chronically dehydrated to one degree or another. Some food consumption surveys indicate that as much as 75 percent of the population (all ages) is chronically mildly dehydrated. Normally, a sensation of thirst manifests after the body has reached a level of dehydration of 0.8 percent to 2 percent loss of body weight. It only takes a small decrease in water to become dehydrated and we often don't respond to thirst by drinking water.

Water can be lost in various ways. Every time you exhale you lose some—as much as two cups a day. Water evaporates invisibly from the surface of your skin too, even when you are not exercising—an additional three cups a day; and each time you urinate you lose even more, probably as much as 6 cups in a 24 hour period. During the course of a normal day a healthy adult can lose about 10 cups of water—and that's before shoveling snow off the sidewalk or working out at the gym. On a hot day, or doing strenuous exercise, you can easily lose up to two gallons (32 cups) of water. If this lost water is not constantly being replenished, you can become seriously dehydrated in no time. This is why we often hear the recommendation of drinking 6 to 8 glasses of water daily. This recommendation is for mild temperatures and low physical activity. In hot or humid weather or when we are engaged in heavy exercise, the body's needs increase—to as much as two gallons a day or more if necessary.

Most of us don't drink the recommended 6 to 8 glasses of water during the day. Many people rely on coffee or soda for their daily fluid

Daily Loss of Water (milliliters)			
	Normal Temperature (68°F/20°C)	Hot Weather	Prolonged Heavy Exercise
Skin	350	350	350
Respiration	350	250	650
Urine	1400	1200	500
Sweat	100	1400	5000
Feces	100	100	100
Total	2300	3300	6600

Source: *Textbook of Medical Physiology, 8th Ed*, Arthur C. Guyton. 1991, W.B. Saunders Company.

allowance. These types of beverages are no substitute for water. They actually have a dehydrating effect so your need for water increases. As a general rule of thumb, for every cup of coffee, tea, or soda you drink, you need to drink at least half that much again in water. So if you drink four cups of coffee per day, you need to drink an additional two cups of plain water to equal the fluid intake you would get from just four cups of water. Alcohol dries up the body big time. For every 1.5 ounces of alcohol you consume, you need to drink an additional 8 ounces of water.

Many drugs can also have a dehydrating effect. Aspirin, ibuprofen, and other non-steroidal anti-inflammatory drugs interfere with kidney function. The same applies to acetaminophen (Tylenol). Antihistamines and some blood pressure medications interfere with heat regulation by decreasing sweating.

Often, we get so busy during the day that we forget to take the time to get a drink. We have to be well on our way toward dehydration before we become uncomfortable enough to get that drink of water. The sensation of thirst is a sign that you are already mildly dehydrated. Ignoring the warning only makes it worse.

The loss of just a small percentage of water can have a significant impact on your health. The early stages of dehydration generally offer no signs or symptoms. You may or may not be thirsty. A loss of just 1 percent of your body weight starts to affect the body's ability to regulate heat and puts stress on the kidneys. Dehydration symptoms generally become noticeable after a loss of 2 percent of normal water volume. Initially, you experience thirst, discomfort, loss of energy, and reduced endurance. At 3 percent, the symptoms become increasingly severe. The heart and respiration rates begin to increase to compensate for decreased plasma volume and lowered blood pressure, while body temperature may rise because of decreased sweating. At 4 percent, headache and dizziness occurs, and physical labor capacity declines by as much as 30 percent. Around 5-6 percent water loss, the body's temperature regulation system starts to fail (sweating has stopped), you experience problems with concentration, drowsiness, nausea, headache, and may feel tingling in the hands or feet. With 8-10 percent fluid loss, muscles may become spastic, skin may shrivel and wrinkle, vision may dim, urination will be greatly reduced and may become painful, and delirium may begin. Eventually the heart cannot beat fast enough to maintain normal blood flow through the body. The pulse becomes weak or cannot be felt, blood pressure falls, and unconsciousness follows. This is circulatory collapse, otherwise known as shock. With water losses greater than 10 percent, damage to the brain, heart, lungs, kidneys, and other organs may occur. At 15 percent you're dead.

Generally, severe dehydration occurs as a result of illness or heavy prolonged exercise. However, mild and moderate dehydration can affect anyone. A useful rule of thumb for avoiding dehydration involves monitoring the frequency and character of urination. If you develop a full bladder at least every 3-4 hours and the urine is clear or only lightly colored, you are likely properly hydrated; if the urine is deeply colored or urination occurs only after several hours or not at all, you are dehydrated. Some nutritional supplements, particularly the B vitamins, will also give urine a darker color. So this test isn't dependable if you are consuming dietary supplements.

While most of us become dehydrated now and again, many are chronically dehydrated. Signs of chronic mild dehydration include dry skin, chapped lips, frequent headaches, constipation, backache, fatigue, and dizziness when standing. Chronic dehydration increases the risk of a number of health problems such as kidney stones, breast cancer, colon cancer, bladder cancer, obesity, mitral valve prolapse (a heart condition), and can adversely affect mental health.[1]

The simple solution is to get into the habit of drinking at least 6 to 8 glasses of water a day. If you drink other beverages, you need to increase your water intake accordingly. Along with water, it would also be a good idea to include a glass or two of coconut water in your daily routine to replenish lost electrolytes. For people who just don't like drinking plain water, coconut water offers an excellent alternative.

DEHYDRATION KILLS

Most of us view dehydration as a minor inconvenience and it may not sound very threatening, but left untreated it can transform into a life-threatening condition. Every summer people fall victim to dehydration caused by heatstroke. Not too long ago the headlines in

Early or mild dehydration:
Thirst
Flushed face
Dry, warm skin
Little or no urine, dark yellow
Dizziness made worse when standing
Weakness
Cramping in the arms and legs
Sleepiness or irritability
Headache
Back pain
Parched and cracked lips
Cracking of the lining of the nose causing the nose to bleed
Dry mouth, dry tongue, thick saliva
Dry and scaly skin

SYMPTOMS OF DEHYDRATION

Moderate to severe dehydration:
Extreme thirst, more than normal or inability to drink
Low blood pressure
Fainting
Severe muscle contractions in the arms, legs, stomach, and back
Lining of the stomach dries out leading to dry heaves and vomiting
Bloated stomach
Sunken fontanelle—soft spot on an infant's head
Sunken dry eyes, with few or no tears
Skin loses its firmness and looks wrinkled or loose
Lack of elasticity of the skin (when a bit of skin is lifted up it stays folded and takes a long time to go back to its normal position)
Rapid and deep breathing
Fast, weak pulse

Severe dehydration:
Above effects become more pronounced
Loss of consciousness, coma
Cool moist extremities
Rapid feeble pulse (the radial pulse may be undetectable)
Very low or undetectable blood pressure
Peripheral cyanosis (extremities display bluish tint caused by lack of circulation)
Major organs, including the heart, lungs, and brain begin to fail

the newspaper described the death of Korey Stringer, a 27-year-old Pro Bowl offensive tackle with the Minnesota Vikings. Stringer died of dehydration and heatstroke after practicing in 90-degree weather. His death came 6 days after University of Florida freshman, Eraste Autin, died from the same condition. Even coaches can fall victim to the heat. During a game Dave Arnold an assistant football coach for Colorado State University collapsed from dehydration on the field and was carried out on a stretcher and taken to the hospital. Athletes and coaches aren't the only ones who suffer from dehydration. In a heat wave that hit the Midwest three residents died in a Detroit nursing home and at least 19 deaths were reported in the Chicago area. Many more occurred in other cities across the country. News stories similar to these repeat themselves every year during the hot summer months.

Dehydration causes millions of deaths worldwide each year. Children are more seriously affected than adults because they become dehydrated more quickly. Dehydration kills more children worldwide than malaria, AIDS, and tuberculosis combined.

Dehydration is a very serious problem in many parts of the world. It is most evident in developing countries where sanitation and hygiene are poor, and infection rates are high. Dehydration accompanies many infectious and food-borne illnesses such as influenza and cholera, which involve fluid loss due to vomiting and diarrhea. About 8,000 children die each day from diarrheal dehydration. Some 3 million people, including 1.9 million children under the age of 5, die each year from diarrhea induced dehydration. Next to pneumonia, dehydration kills more children worldwide than any other illness. Even in the United States where health care is readily available, about 1,000 children die each year from dehydration.

The most common cause of dehydration is due to illnesses caused by rotavirus, E. coli, shigella, campylobacter, salmonella, and epidemics of cholera. Of these, rotavirus is by far the most widespread. Rotavirus causes profuse vomiting, diarrhea, and dehydration. The primary cause of death in many illnesses, such as rotavirus and cholera, is not from the disease itself, but from dehydration. If the patient can be kept hydrated, symptoms lessen, and chances for survival improve immensely. Rotavirus is so contagious and resilient that almost every child worldwide will be infected by it at least once before he or she is five years old.

The incidence is nearly the same in industrialized countries like the US as it is in developing countries. In poor countries rotavirus kills about 600,000 children a year.

Dehydration can also occur if you do not eat or drink much during an illness. Nausea or mouth sores, for example, make drinking less desirable. Some medications can make the situation worse by promoting water loss.

Dehydration isn't just a consequence of illness or drugs. It can happen anytime, anywhere, to anybody. It is very common when the climate is hot, humid, or when someone engages in heavy physical activity. Simply not drinking enough water can cause it. So can the consumption of excessive amounts of alcohol without adequate water.

ORAL REHYDRATION THERAPY

Since dehydration is caused by a loss of water from the body, the logical solution is simply drink more water. In mild cases, this is all that is generally needed. However, in moderate and severe cases, drinking water is not enough, and in some cases may make the situation even worse.

Dehydration can occur any time fluid loss exceeds the amount the body absorbs. The digestive tract can only absorb so much water at a time. When a large amount of water is consumed, much of it rushes though the digestive tract without being absorbed. So drinking a lot of water won't necessarily replenish the amount lost.

Another complication is that dehydration involves more than just fluid loss. When water exits the body, it takes along with it mineral salts or electrolytes such as sodium and potassium. This can quickly deplete the body's electrolytes. A drop in electrolytes is just as serious as the lack of water. Dehydration involves the loss of both water and electrolytes. If just water is given to a person suffering from dehydration, the situation may get worse because this water will dilute the remaining electrolytes in the body, causing a greater mineral deficiency. However, even if electrolytes are added to the water, the body may not be able to absorb the solution fast enough to replenish fluid and electrolytes lost.

In the 1960s acute diarrhea was killing around 5 million children worldwide each year, mostly in developing countries. Giving the children water to drink did not work because the liquid rushed though the digestive tract too quickly to be absorbed by body tissues. The only answer seemed to be to bypass the digestive system and rehydrate the body using intravenous therapy. This is an invasive and traumatic procedure for a child. Since it must be administered by someone with medical training, it was impractical for most cases of childhood diarrhea since most of those who needed it did not have access to medical attention.

In 1968 researchers in India discovered that adding glucose and salt to water in the right proportions enabled the liquid to be absorbed faster through the intestinal wall. Glucose's chemical properties allow mineral salts to be absorbed more efficiently. The salt then promotes the absorption of water into the capillaries within the intestinal wall, which carry the water and electrolytes to other parts of the body and restore fluid balance. So anyone suffering from diarrhea could replace the lost fluids and salts simply by drinking the solution. That discovery was called oral rehydration therapy (ORT). ORT had the potential to save the lives of millions of people. Although this simple treatment initially faced resistance from the medical community, it was eventually described in the prestigious British medical journal *The Lancet* (Aug 5, 1978) as "potentially the most important medical advance of this century."

In the early 1900s cholera epidemics swept the Indian subcontinent. Death from cholera is caused primarily by diarrhea-induced dehydration. Fluid loss from diarrhea occurs so rapidly that its victims can die within four to eight hours or, as lore has it, "before they can dig their own graves." The only effective treatment at the time was intravenous therapy. Consequently, millions who did not have access to proper medical care died. Vaccines to treat cholera had never been completely effective. In 1960 a cholera research laboratory was established in Bangladesh. Its mission was to evaluate treatments for cholera. In the late 1960s they began experimenting with ORT and achieved remarkable success. Fatalities among diarrhea patients at the facility dropped from 50 percent to zero—quite an amazing success rate!

Despite their astonishing success, they faced resistance from the medical profession, particularly in the West, who dismissed this simple remedy as inferior to the standard and much costlier IV therapy. This initial reluctance by the medical establishment prevented the therapy from gaining acceptance and the recognition it deserved. If it wasn't for an upheaval in the political environment at the time, it probably would have taken decades for it to gain acceptance in mainstream medicine. Ironically, it took a war and the deaths of thousands of people to prove to the world the effectiveness of oral rehydration therapy.

The opportunity came in 1971 during Bangladesh's war for independence from Pakistan. In a mass exodus nine million refugees streamed across the boarder into India. Cholera broke out in the refugee camps. Dilip Mahalanabis, MD, an Indian physician who had participated in the oral rehydration studies, brought in a medical team from Calcutta to treat the disease. His team began using the standard IV treatment, but within weeks, his supplies were exhausted.

Amid the awful scenes of people suffering and dying, Dr. Mahalanabis, out of sheer desperation, began administering ORT. With the aid of volunteers, oral rehydration fluids were prepared and disseminated to the thousands who were sick. One of the primary objections of using ORT voiced by the medical community was that if the solution was not prepared or administered properly by trained medical personnel, it might kill more people than it saved. Despite the fact that lay people performed most of the work in the camps, the fatality rate dropped from 30 percent to just 3 percent. The gamble paid off and proved beyond doubt the effectiveness of ORT.

Afterwards skepticism among the medical profession continued. Medical journals refused to publish Mahalanabis' paper about the success of ORT during the outbreak. Fortunately, Mahalanabis gained an ally in Dhiman Barua, then head of the World Health Organization's bacterial diseases unit in Geneva, Switzerland and a survivor of a massive cholera epidemic that occurred in Bangladesh in 1932. Barua visited the refugee camps during the crisis and saw firsthand the effectiveness of the therapy. Realizing its potential, he pushed for the acceptance of ORT in all of the United Nations health agencies. "The simplicity and power of this tool give it its own momentum," Mahalanabis said.

Oral rehydration treatment can reverse dehydration in more than 90 percent of patients, even in cases of severe diarrhea caused by rotavirus and cholera. Today, at least 2 million lives are saved each year through ORT.

Despite the success, millions of people continue to die each year from dehydration. In parts of Asia and Africa the fight against diarrhea is hampered by the lack of clean water and poor sanitary conditions. In countries like Ethiopia, only 40 percent of the population has access to safe water, and fewer than 1 in 3 has regular access to sanitary toilet facilities, which at a minimum means a pit latrine. Most rural Ethiopians don't make the connection between the way they dispose of human waste and their family's health. As a consequence, the average Ethiopian child suffers five to 12 episodes of diarrhea a year. During the rainy season the problem is worse because sewage seeps into water supplies. In Ethiopia between 50,000 and 112,000 children under 5 die from diarrhea every year. Infants perish because they don't live near a hospital or parents don't know about or how to administer oral rehydration therapy themselves. (For information on treating dehydration at home see "Guide to Giving Oral Rehydration Therapy at Home" in the Appendix.)

Mild dehydration can be treated simply by drinking additional water; more serious cases require special fluids with an isotonic mixture of water, salt, and sugar. The World Health Organization (WHO) has developed a powdered solution packaged in little pouches which they disseminate to hospitals throughout the world. All a person has to do is add a liter of clean water. One of the drawbacks is not having packets available when needed. If a parent doesn't have it available, he or she must seek medical assistance. Another drawback is price. Although to most of us, the cost would seem small, it may be more expensive than some can afford so they don't have it on hand when needed. Palatability is another factor. The high salt content makes the solution a bit difficult to swallow. But, the reasoning is that if a person is seriously dehydrated, they will drink just about anything to quench their thirst.

Nature has provided us with perhaps a better solution, a natural rehydration beverage in the form of coconut water. In many parts of the world seriously affected by dehydration, coconuts grow in abundance. Coconut palms produce fruit all year round so they are always available and in many cases free for the picking. This provides people a rehydration fluid that is cheap, easy to get, readily available, and tastes good. A child is more likely to drink the sweet liquid from a fresh coconut than a salty chemical solution.

The obvious advantages of using coconut water as a means of ORT was recognized soon after the Bangladesh experience. It had proven to be successful as an intravenous rehydration solution. Why not use it for the same purpose orally? It was already a popular beverage and readily accepted by people in many parts of the world.

THE COCONUT WATER SOLUTION

In the coconut growing regions of the world, coconut and its products hold a high place of respect among the locals. Its oil, meat, water, and milk are used for food and for medicine. It is not surprising to learn that in some communities coconut water is prized for its rejuvenating powers. In Nigeria, for instance, among coastal dwellers it has a long tradition of use as a remedy for diarrhea and dehydration.[2] Unfortunately, most people are unaware of this traditional remedy, especially those who live inland away from the ocean or in environments where coconuts don't normally grow.

Outbreaks of cholera in Africa and in the Pacific Islands during the 1970s prompted increased interest in the use of coconut water as an oral rehydration fluid.[3] In cases where coconut water was used, survival rates were encouraging. Sadly however, many children died while coconuts, a potential cure, stood untouched just feet away.

Researchers compared the nutritional makeup of coconut water with oral rehydration solution which had been proven to be effective in treating cholera induced dehydration.[4-5] Coconut water was found to be superior in every aspect to sodas, fruit juices, and other common beverages for rehydration. However, prejudice against the use of coconut water was strong. Many expressed concern about its relatively low sodium content. It was suggested that simply adding table salt to the coconut water would make up for this apparent deficiency.[6] Salt is readily available and can be easily added to coconut water or added to foods given in conjunction with the water. In an emergency situation where medical help or commercial oral rehydration solution is not available, this combination would provide a suitable solution even in serious situations such as a cholera epidemic. A thumb and two finger pinch of salt to a liter of coconut water was suggested as a means to increase sodium content to match that in commercial ORT solutions.

Researchers at the University of the Philippines PGH Medical Center attempted to improve on nature and transform coconut water into an "ideal" oral rehydration fluid.[7] This improved fluid was called "modified coconut water." Water from a young coconut was diluted with distilled water in a 1:1 ratio to reduce the potassium concentration by half and to raise the pH to neutral. To every liter of the diluted coconut water, 1 gram of sodium chloride, 2.5 grams of sodium bicarbonate, and 15 grams of glucose were added. These adjustments gave the coconut water a similar profile to commercial rehydration solutions, but with the added benefit of all the other nutrients naturally found in the water.

Fifty-eight infants and children, aged 3 months to 6 years, were chosen to test the new solution. Each were suffering from acute diarrhea with mild to moderate dehydration. Patients were given between 100 to 200 ml (3.4-6.8 oz) of modified coconut water over a 24 hour period. No food or other therapeutic aid was given except for the water. Significant improvement was noted in 43 (74.14 percent) of the patients with no adverse effects. This study proved that "modified" coconut water was safe and effective.

In 1990 British researchers in India compared coconut water to the standard WHO oral rehydration salt (ORS) solution in the treatment of cholera-induced dehydration.[8] To the surprise of everyone, coconut water, *without modification*, improved total fluid retention significantly better than the ORS solution.

Could a natural product be better than a scientifically designed formula? This didn't sit well with some in the medical community.

Two years later another study by researchers in the West Indies demonstrated that fresh coconut water can be successfully used as a home treatment for dehydration.[9] Again, without modification, coconut water proved to be an effective oral rehydration solution. Despite its success, however, the medical profession was resistant to the idea of using the juice from coconuts to treat a medical problem. Even the authors of this study expressed caution in using coconut water in severe cases of dehydration or when kidney function was impaired.

The medical establishment continued to resist the idea that coconut water could be as effective as the more costly and "scientifically" formulated ORS. In an attempt to discredit and discourage the use of coconut water for rehydration, another study was published a year later.[10]

In this study the authors did a chemical analysis on the electrolyte content of coconut water at various stages of development. Their findings showed—as had already been reported in previous studies—that at all stages of growth the electrolyte concentration of coconut water was higher in potassium and lower in sodium and chloride than blood plasma and ORS solution. Based on their analysis, they "theorized" that coconut water was useless as an oral rehydration fluid. In fact, they expressed concern that it might even be harmful. As preposterous as it may sound, the authors warned that coconut water consumption may be dangerous if used as a rehydration beverage.

In their haste to condemn coconut water, however, the authors apparently didn't bother to do their homework. If they had, they would have found studies reporting the successful treatment of dehydration using both fresh coconut and modified coconut water. This study completely debunked the use of coconut water solely on its sodium and potassium content without evaluating it in a clinical setting. The recommendation of this study goes contrary to several previous studies and to clinical experiences reported in the Philippines, Oceania, and the Caribbean where health care workers had been using coconut water successfully to combat diarrheal dehydration for over a decade.

In a letter published in the prestigious medical journal *The Lancet,* Dr. E.S. Cooper from the Gloucestershire Royal Hospital in the UK responded to the critics.[11] "I must feel some concern when [critics] say that the electrolyte composition of this fluid makes it potentially dangerous for children with acute diarrhea." He goes on to say it is no more dangerous than "boiled water." If anyone should know, it was Cooper. His knowledge wasn't based on a theory, but actual experience. For ten years beginning in the mid 1970s he had worked on the Caribbean island of St. Lucia. While he was there, he encouraged the use of coconut water for the treatment of diarrhea and dehydration. Coconut water was so effective that the people began to believe it could cure just about anything and it became a part of the folklore of the island.

The success and efficiency of coconut water as a rehydration fluid has been proven time and time again around the world in various situations. This was very clearly demonstrated recently by the tsunami victims who survived for weeks and even months with no water or fluids to drink whatsoever except for coconut water. Coconut water did not dehydrate them, it saved them from dehydration, thus putting to rest the fears of the critics. Theories don't mean anything if they are proven wrong by real life experience. Actual use and clinical studies have proven coconut water to be highly effective as a rehydration fluid.

Researchers later discovered that ORS solutions containing less sodium worked better than the standard solutions.[12] The risk of requiring intravenous infusion after initial oral rehydration declined when children were given reduced sodium solution. It was discovered that too much sodium in the fluid often led to hypernatremia (high blood sodium), a potentially fatal condition. The sodium content in coconut water would not cause a sodium overload.

Despite initial reluctance from the medical community, today physicians and researchers who work with dehydration victims along with several international organizations such as The Food and Agricultural Organization and the World Health Organization have recognized young coconut water as a useful home treatment for diarrhea induced dehydration.[13-16]

A NATURAL SPORTS DRINK

Clinical studies and actual experience have demonstrated that young coconut water can be a useful aid in the fight against diarrhea induced dehydration. The next question: is it of value in combating dehydration caused by other means such as excessive heat and strenuous exercise? The answer is a definite "Yes."

The effectiveness of young coconut water as a sports rehydration fluid was demonstrated in a comprehensive study published in the *Journal of Physiological Anthropology and Applied Human Science* in 2002.[17]

Eight healthy college-age subjects were chosen to participate in this study. They engaged in strenuous exercise (running on a treadmill) in a hot environment to induce dehydration. Subjects lost on average 2.78 percent of their body weight in water during the activity. They were allowed to rest for 30 minutes without drinking anything. They were then given one of three beverages and monitored over the next two hours to evaluate the effectiveness of the beverages in rehydration. The beverages were plain water, young coconut water, and a commercial rehydration solution. They were allowed to drink a precise amount at three intervals during the 2-hour rehydration period. The study was

No Trip to the Hospital this Time!

Several years ago I somehow got achalasia (a disorder of the esophagus that interferes with swallowing). It began with not being able to keep food down and when I could no longer keep liquids down within a few weeks I was hospitalized for dehydration. I needed electrolytes desperately but couldn't keep anything down long enough to extract them. The doctors almost demanded I have surgery, but I refused believing there had to be another way. Fortunately, I found an article on the web that allowed me to manage the disease with moderate success.

Four days ago without notice I found myself in the same boat not being able to keep anything down—neither food nor liquid. I had lost about 17 lbs in the past four days and was going down fast. Not being willing to accept this as fact, I went to the web again. This time God directed me (and I don't say this lightly) to your website (www.coconutresearchcenter.org). I KNOW it was Him. I read your words like a sponge. I feverishly researched how to get the electrolytes that my body would accept. After reading about young coconut juice on your site, I called a friend of mine who owns a successful Asian market in Boston, where my wife and I reside. I immediately bought a case of sixty small containers of the frozen fresh juice and MIRACULOUSLY this morning was able to drink eight of them. The first one went down and about 10 percent stayed down. The second one I kept about 20 percent down. By the eighth one I was able to swallow and keep the entire thing down. I drank about 10 more during the day and they have all stayed down. It is truly a miracle. I am far from over the loss of energy from my acute symptoms and resulting effects over the last four days but as of tonight, I can tell I am 90 percent better and there will be no trip to the hospital. IT'S WORKING!!

S. W.

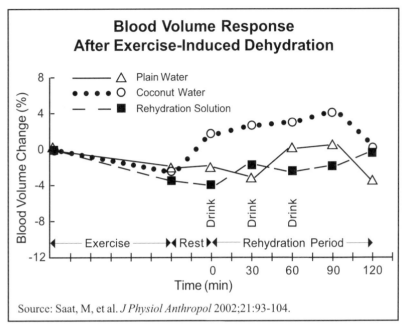

Blood volume response after exercise-induced dehydration and during the 2 hour rehydration period.

repeated weekly over a three week period so that each subject had a turn drinking each of the three beverages.

All three beverages were useful in rehydrating the subjects under the conditions tested and most of the parameters evaluated were similar. However, coconut water had the most dramatic effect on restoring blood volume. Fluid loss was restored to the blood almost immediately upon consuming the coconut water. Total fluid volume actually increased by about 4 percent above pre-exercise levels and remained elevated for about 90 minutes until tapering off to pre-exercise levels at the end of the two hour rest period (see graph above).

The oral rehydration solution replenished blood volume slowly and did not restore pre-exercise levels until the very end of the 2-hour rest period. Plain water restored pre-exercise blood volume levels in about 1 hour, but actually lost volume by the end of the 2-hour rest period.

Judging from this data, coconut water is superior to plain water and oral rehydration solution for restoring lost water to the bloodstream.

While some researchers have expressed concern about the potassium and sodium concentrations in young coconut water, it apparently had no harmful effect. Indeed, the coconut water appears to work better than plain water and the scientifically formulated oral rehydration solution. We know from the studies mentioned in the previous chapter that when coconut water is injected directly into the bloodstream it does not upset potassium and sodium balance. So that is a non-issue.

Researchers also evaluated how the subjects felt during the rehydration period. The sensation of nausea and upset stomach often experienced after drinking other beverages was significantly lower when they drank coconut water. In addition, the subjects could drink all of the coconut water provided to them without adverse effects, while it took longer to drink the other beverages.

The mild sweetness and palatability of the coconut water made it easier and more enjoyable to consume despite its high electrolyte content. Throughout the study the subjects found that consuming the plain water and the rehydration solution reduced their stimulus to drink. In one case, plain water caused nausea and some subjects vomited, and the trial had to be repeated on another day.

Palatability determines to a great extent the amount of fluid people will drink even if they are dehydrated.[18] People are more likely to consume enough coconut water to adequately rehydrate themselves. However, they may not consume enough water or rehydration solution to reach pre-exercise hydration levels. The researchers concluded that considering all of the characteristics of coconut water, it makes an "ideal" rehydration fluid.

Why does coconut water restore water volume better than other fluids? Apparently it has to do with the electrolyte balance in our bodies. Our bodies are made up of about 60 percent water. Twenty percent is extracellular fluid (the fluid outside the cells), this includes blood plasma 4 percent and interstitial fluid (fluid surrounding our cells) 16 percent. The remaining 40 percent of body water is intracellular fluid—the fluid inside our cells. So we have twice as much fluid inside our cells as we do outside.

Extracellular fluid (outside the cell) is high in sodium and low in potassium. Intracellular fluid (inside the cell) is just the opposite being high in potassium and low in sodium. The electrolyte content of coconut water is more like intracellular than extracellular fluid, yet still somewhat like both. Thus it provides elements essential for replenishing both fluids, including many trace minerals which are also lost in perspiration.

When we perspire, plasma (extracellular fluid) volume decreases first because it provides the precursor fluid for perspiration. However, water loss from exercise and heat is derived from *both* intracellular and extracellular fluids.[19] Within the first 10-15 minutes of strenuous exercise plasma is reduced by 5-15 percent. If exercise continues beyond this, water loss continues due to sweating, but there is little further change in the plasma volume in the absence of fluid intake. Plasma volume is maintained by drawing fluid from inside the cells. The cells of the body can become very dehydrated. When fluids are consumed

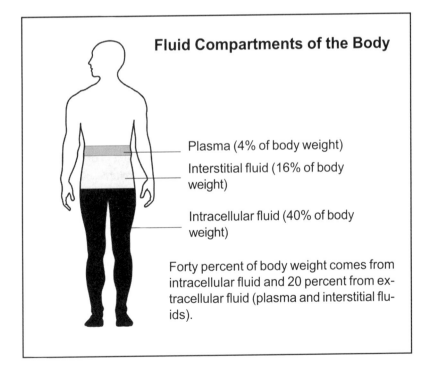

Fluid Compartments of the Body

Plasma (4% of body weight)

Interstitial fluid (16% of body weight)

Intracellular fluid (40% of body weight)

Forty percent of body weight comes from intracellular fluid and 20 percent from extracellular fluid (plasma and interstitial fluids).

and the body is rehydrated, there is a greater tendency for the body to restore intracellular fluid first.[20]

As fluids are lost, both sodium and potassium are depleted. Potassium is important because it is the primary electrolyte in intracellular fluid. Dehydration depletes the cells of this important element. Because of coconut water's unique chemistry it appears to restore both extracellular and intracellular fluid in a highly efficient manner, making it an ideal sports drink.

COMMERCIAL SPORTS DRINKS

Sports drinks are a familiar sight to us all. Amateur and professional athletes as well as ordinary consumers guzzle them down by the quart. Sports drinks have become a multimillion dollar business with numerous brands to choose from.

The very first sports drink was formulated by researchers at the University of Florida in an effort to help the then struggling Florida Gators football team. In 1965 the Gators coach asked university physicians for help in finding a solution to the dehydration and fatigue that plagued the players. In games and on the practice field players were wilting in the hot, humid Florida climate.

The researchers set to work and developed a new beverage that would replace the fluids and electrolytes lost in sweat and provide ample carbohydrates (sugar) to sustain energy. They called the new drink "Gatorade" after the school's mascot the Florida Gator. The new drink helped counteract debilitating dehydration far better than plain water, giving the Gators the stamina they needed to outlast their opponents. Fueled by Gatorade the Gators finished the 1966 season with a 7-4 record—their first winning season in a decade. The following year they went 9-2, and won the Orange Bowl for the first time in school history.

Word of the Gators success using the new sports drink spread and other universities began ordering it for their teams. Gatorade gained national attention in 1969 when it was adopted by Kansas City Chiefs. In that year the Chiefs went 11-3 winning the AFL championship and ended the season with a stunning 23-7 victory over the heavily favored NFL champion Minnesota Vikings in Super Bowl IV.

Gatorade was launched as a sports drink for the public in 1968. It is now distributed by PepsiCo. The original beverage was not like the commercial product you see on the store shelves today. Because of its high electrolyte content, it had a strong salty taste that even the sugar couldn't tame. When it was marketed to consumers, the formula was watered down to reduce the electrolyte content. Sugar was increased and flavorings added to make the drink more appealing to customers. The new drink was more of a non-carbonated soft drink than a serious rehydration fluid.

The popularity of Gatorade spurred the sports drink phenomenon and the introduction of numerous other sports beverages. Gatorade is the standard by which all other sports drinks are compared. Let's take a look at the contents of Gatorade and compare it with coconut water.

The ingredients label on Gatorade Original Orange lists: water, sucrose syrup, high fructose corn syrup, citric acid, natural orange flavor with other natural flavors, salt, sodium citrate, monopotassium phosphate, yellow 6, glycerol ester of wood rosin, and brominated vegetable oil.

The three main ingredients are water, sugar (sucrose syrup), and sugar (glucose-fructose syrup). So it is mostly sugar water. Despite the claim of "natural orange flavor and other natural flavors," it contains no fruit juice. These "natural" flavors could be just about anything and may be as far from being natural as turpentine. The US Code of Federal Regulations states that natural flavorings include "...essential oil, oleoresin, essence or extractive, protein hydrolysate, distillate, or any distillate, or any products of roasting, heating or enzymolysis, which contains the flavoring constituents derived from a spice, fruit or fruit juice, vegetable or vegetable juice, edible yeast, herb, bark, bud, root, leaf or similar plant material, meat, seafood, poultry, eggs, dairy products, or fermentation products thereof, whose significant function in food is flavoring rather than nutritional." Hmm...so it contains some of this stuff, whatever it is.

The next ingredient is salt. Salt, of course, is sodium chloride. This is basically the sole source of electrolytes in the beverage. All the other chemical additives listed are there for taste, texture, and stability.

Contrary to what some people believe, sodium citrate and monopotassium phosphate are not there as a source of electrolytes. Sodium citrate is a flavor enhancer and preservative. Monopotassium phosphate is a multipurpose chemical which is used by industries as a fungicide, fertilizer, and food additive. It is added to foods as a buffering agent to balance pH. The most common consumer uses are in cigarettes and Gatorade.

Yellow 6 is a chemical dye used to give the beverage an appealing color. The FDA describes yellow 6 as "the disodium salt of 6-hydroxy-5-[(4-sulfophenyl)azo]-2-naphthalenesulfonic acid." Yummm, doesn't that sound appetizing? No wonder they just call it "Yellow 6." The thought of consuming anything that sounds like it belongs in a can of paint thinner or diesel fuel is a little disconcerting.

Ester gum or *glycerol ester of wood rosin* as it is also called, is used as a stabilizer to keep oils in suspension in water. It is used in making varnish, soap, and soldering flux as well as an additive in foods.

The most troubling ingredient listed is brominated vegetable oil, which is vegetable oil that is chemically bonded to the element bromine. Brominated vegetable oil is an emulsifier used in citrus flavored drinks to help flavors stay suspended and produce the cloudy appearance characteristic of Gatorade. Bromine is a halogen that blocks iodine utilization in the thyroid and other tissues in the body. Long after consumption, traces remain in the body. Adverse reactions have been reported from the consumption of beverages containing brominated vegetable oil. These reactions include fatigue, headaches, tremors, memory loss, hallucinations, and seizures.

A case documented in the *Journal of Toxicology* illustrates the potential danger of drinking beverages containing this substance. A man who had been drinking about three liters of soda daily was admitted to the hospital emergency room with confusion, headaches, tremors, and memory loss. His right eyelid drooped uncontrollably down over his eye. Doctors suspected some type of brain damage. His condition deteriorated over the next 30 days as doctors tried to determine what was wrong. During his stay he lost the ability to walk and was pretty much down for the count. Eventually, the doctors identified the problem as bromism and six hours of hemodialysis pulled him through. Since bromine collects in body tissues, even the 30 day stay in the hospital without the beverage wasn't enough to flush it from his system. His health continued to decline until he was diagnosed and given proper treatment.[21] If you are a serious athlete drinking a lot of fluids you need a beverage that is going to support your health and not destroy it. Although Gatorade is used in our example here, all commercial sports drinks are essentially the same. They are mostly sugar water with a little salt and a lot of questionable additives.

Now let's take a look at coconut water. The ingredients in coconut water are 100 percent all natural with no preservatives, artificial colors, additives, sugars, chemicals, or artificial anything. It is a "living" food with a natural combination of easily absorbable electrolytes, sugars, amino acids, vitamins, and other nutrients. No harmful effects have ever been reported with drinking coconut water, even in large amounts. From a health and nutritional standpoint, there is no comparison between coconut water and commercial sports drinks.

Amino Acid Content of Coconut Water

Amino Acid	mg/100g	mg/cup
Tryptophan	8	19
Threonine	26	62
Isoleucine	28	67
Leucine	53	127
Lysine	32	77
Methionine	13	31
Cystine	14	34
Phenylalanine	37	89
Tyrosine	22	53
Valine	44	106
Arginine	118	283
Histidine	17	41
Alanine	37	89
Aspartic acid	70	168
Glutamic acid	165	396
Glycine	34	82
Proline	30	72
Serine	37	89

Source: USDA National Nutrient Database for Standard Reference (2006).

Coconut water contains 18 amino acids. Sports drinks contain none.

Nutrient Content in Gatorade, Powerade, and Coconut Water (Value per 100 grams)

Nutrient	Units	Gatorade	Powerade	Coconut Water*
Sugar	g	5.33	6.02	3.71
Dietary fiber	g	0	0	1.1
Calcium	mg	1	2	24
Iron	mg	0.20	0.25	0.29
Magnesium	mg	1	5	25
Phosphorous	mg	9	2	20
Potassium	mg	14	13	250
Sodium	mg	39	22	105
Zinc	mg	0.26	0.06	0.10
Copper	mg	0.25	0.25	0.04
Manganese	mg	0.05	0.05	0.142
Selenium	mcg	0.0	0.0	1
Fluoride	mcg	34	62	trace
Vitamin C	mg	0.4	0.4	2.4
Thiamin	mg	0.011	0.011	0.030
Niacin	mg	0.22	1.54	0.08
Pantothenic acid	mg	0.055	0.055	0.043
Vitamin B-6	mg	0.022	0.153	0.032
Folate	mcg	0.0	0.0	3
Amino acids	mg	0.0	0.0	785

*Unlike commercially produced beverages, natural products like coconut water do not have a precise chemical profile. All values listed here are averages of samples tested. These values will vary somewhat due to age, variety, and growing conditions.
Source: USDA National Nutrient Database for Standard Reference (2006).

Gatorade's biggest rival is Powerade by Coca-Cola. The chart above compares the nutrient content of these sports drinks with coconut water. This data comes out of the USDA National Nutrient Database, so we can assume the information is accurate. According to these figures coconut water contains more minerals and nutrients and significantly less sugar than either sports drink. There is one ingredient, however, that is significantly higher in Gatorade and Powerade than in coconut water and that is fluoride. The fluoride comes from fluoridated tap water used in the manufacturing of these beverages. Coconut water has only trace amounts of fluoride, as it should be with all trace minerals in our foods.

There is another very interesting feature. Take a look at the sodium content of each of the beverages. Notice that both sports drinks have only a fraction as much as coconut water. Ironically, the low sodium content of coconut water was the reason why it was criticized as not being an ideal rehydration fluid; however, it contains more than twice as much as Gatorade. As a serious rehydration beverage Gatorade and Powerade do not compare to coconut water. If you are physically active and perspire a lot, coconut water is by far a better choice. This is particularly true if you are a serious athlete.

Most sports drinks are nothing more than soft drinks loaded with sugar and artificial additives and shy on electrolytes and nutrients. Their effect on rehydrating the body is only minimal. Coconut water, on the other hand, has proven itself useful in both intravenous and oral rehydration therapy for mild and serious cases of dehydration. It is sweet and refreshing with less sugar and no chemical additives, thus making it one of, if not the best, sports rehydration beverages you can drink.

Hypothetically, if you became seriously dehydrated and required intravenous fluids but your only choice for rehydration was either coconut water or Gatorade, which one would you choose? I can't imagine the damage Gatorade might cause if it was pumped directly into the bloodstream. However, coconut water has been proven safe. The purpose of drinking fluids in a dehydration situation is to replenish what has been removed from the blood and other compartments of the body. So why would you want to replace it with something that is not completely compatible with the body?

EXERCISE-INDUCED DEHYDRATION

When I was involved in school sports in the 1960s, we were advised not to drink too much water during practice because it would cause stomach cramps. Even though we were working out in 90 plus degree temperatures and sweating profusely, we drank as little water as possible during practice. Today we know this idea to be false, and actually harmful. An athlete needs to replenish liquids as quickly as possible.

Anybody can fall victim to dehydration, even competitive athletes who are well aware of its dangers. Shanna learned this the hard way. She was a well conditioned athlete competing in a one half Ironman triathlon. It turned out to be a very hot west Texas day, with temperatures soaring above 100 degrees F (38 C). She had raced in the heat before so was no stranger to hot weather. Problems started almost from the start. After only one mile, she started experiencing diarrhea and painful leg cramps. By mile 6½ her head ached and she stopped sweating. She managed a slow, painful finish, tried to rehydrate herself, but became delirious. The medical staff was called. Intravenous fluids were started, but her condition deteriorated and she began vomiting. After being transferred to the hospital, she began to have seizures. She experienced widespread muscle breakdown, severe electrolyte disturbance, kidney damage, and her lungs filled with fluid. She was placed on artificial life support and was given a 50 percent chance of survival. Fortunately, she lived.

If a well trained athlete, who is very aware of the dangers of dehydration, can fall victim, so can you and I. While we may not participate in a triathlon or marathon, water loss on a hot day with moderate activity can be enough to cause serious harm.

Humidity as well as heat can be a problem. The purpose of sweat is to cool the body and prevent overheating. When sweat evaporates, it carries off heat, which in turn, keeps us cool. In humid conditions the rate of sweating is higher and cooling is less effective because the air is already saturated with water and sweat can't evaporate. Sweat that doesn't evaporate doesn't contribute to the cooling process. However, sweat does deplete the body of vital water and salt. As dehydration progresses, cooling becomes more difficult. Performance drops and heat injury becomes a real threat. Air temperatures don't have to be high for dehydration to occur. Deaths have occurred when the temperature was less than 75 degrees F (24 C) but the relative humidity was above 95 percent.

It may seem obvious to drink during heavy physical activity, but many people underestimate the magnitude of their fluid loss. It is very difficult to avoid dehydration during a long race or when working in the

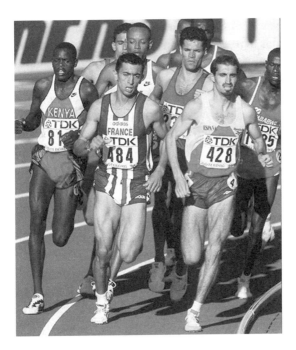

Many amateur and professional athletes are using coconut water to improve hydration and optimize performance.

heat because the rate of sweat loss usually exceeds the rate of absorption of ingested fluids. The maximum rate of fluid absorption by the gastrointestinal tract during exercise is approximately 800 ml (27 ounces) per hour. The rate of fluid loss through sweating can easily reach 1 liter (34 ounces) per hour and can soar to 2 liters per hour under very strenuous conditions. Thus, it is not possible to drink enough to stay hydrated and, dehydration will still occur despite drinking plenty of fluid.

Drinking a lot of water can cause discomfort and bloating. So guzzling a liter of water every hour will not replenish the lost liquids and may make you feel sick. Also, realize that the more dehydrated you get, the harder it is for your digestive tract to absorb what you drink. If you work out heavily in a hot environment, no amount of water is going to keep you hydrated.

In addition to a need to replenish lost water, you must also replenish lost electrolytes. An electrolyte deficiency can be just as dangerous as a water deficiency. Drinking only water, without a source of electrolytes, can dilute the remaining electrolytes in your bloodstream causing hyponatermia—low blood sodium. Electrolyte deficiency can cause severe reactions, which can send you to the hospital or even worse.

The following illustrates this point. Triathlons are endurance races that include swimming, cycling, and running. Short races can be completed in less then 1½ hours, longer races may last 12 hours or more. Immediately following a short triathlon a competitor collapsed. He was rushed to the emergency room, vomiting and in extreme pain. He was suffering from hyponatremia, believed to be caused by vomiting, induced by dehydration. The emergency room physician encouraged him to drink more water during his races to stay hydrated. He was a well conditioned "front of the pack" level triathlete and consistently finished in the top 10 percent. So he was very accustomed to hard exercise and competition. Following the physician's advice, he drank more water at his next race, but ended up back in the emergency room. The medical staff eventually realized that the cause for his visits to the hospital weren't because he was not drinking enough water, it was because he was drinking too much water without supplying the needed electrolytes.

During exercise in the heat, more salt is lost in sweat per hour than is usually replaced by food and fluid or by commercial sports drinks. This triathlete began drinking beverages containing the needed electrolytes before and after his races. He is now able to train and race under a wide variety of conditions and has not had a further episode.

Many athletes who rely solely on water or sports drinks for hydration are to some level hyponatremic. It is estimated that up to 30 percent of the finishers of the Hawaiian Ironman Triathlon are both dehydrated and hyponatremic. Ultradistance athletes have a similar track record.

Sweat contains between 2.25-3.40 grams of salt (sodium chloride) per liter, and the rate of perspiration during strenuous exercise can easily average 1 liter per hour. Experts recommend that during a long, hot race, you should aim for a total sodium intake of about 1 gram per hour. To get 1 gram (1000 mg) of sodium into your body, you would need to drink two and a half liters (84 ounces) of Gatorade—certainly impractical every hour! To get 1 gram of sodium from table salt, you would need to ingest 2.5 grams (1 gram from sodium plus 1.5 grams for chloride). A teaspoon of salt weights approximately 6.6 grams. So

FLUID BALANCE TEST

How much fluid should you drink while exercising? Individuals vary widely in their net water loss while exercising in the heat, dependent upon sweat rate, rate of fluid ingestion, rate of gastric emptying, type of fluid ingested, percentage body fat, and other variables. The amount of fluids you need will be different from that of someone else. The following test allows you to determine exactly how much dehydration you incur during your workout so that you know how much lost water you need to replace. Results will vary depending on the temperature, so you may want to repeat this test often.

1. Empty your bladder and record your weight (nude or swim suit).
Pre-exercise weight = _(A)_ lbs.

2. Do your usual workout, and drink as you normally would.

3. Record the volume of fluid you consume during exercise.
How much you drank = _____ fluid ounces.

4. Towel dry, empty your bladder and then record your weight (nude or swim suit).
Post-exercise weight = _(B)_ lbs.

5. Subtract your post-exercise weight from your pre-exercise weight to get the number of pounds you lost during exercise.
A – B = _(C)_ lbs.

6. To find out how many fluid ounces of water you have lost, multiply C by 15.3.
C x 15.3 = _____ fluid ounces of water you lost during exercise.

7. To find out what percentage of your weight you lost during exercise divide (C) by (A) and multiply by 100.
(C / A) x 100 = _____ % body weight lost.

Metric units. To calculate water loss in milliliters, use kilograms for A, B, and C and multiply C by 995.34 in Step 6.

Example
Pre-exercise weight: 160 lbs.
Amount of fluids consumed: 12 ounces
Post-exercise weight: 158 lbs.
Weight lost: 160 lbs. − 158 lbs. = 2 lbs
Amount of water lost: 2 lbs. x 15.3 = 30.6 ounces
Percentage of body weight lost: (158/160) x 100 = 1.25%

Total percent of body weight lost during the workout is 1.25%. Compare this to the figures in the table below to gauge degree of dehydration. This number indicates mild dehydration. Consumption of an additional 30.6 ounces of fluid (a total of 42.6 ounces) is needed to achieve zero fluid loss.

0% — normal heat regulation and performance
1% — thirst is stimulated, heat regulation during exercise is altered, performance begins to decline
2% — further decrease in heat regulation, increased thirst, worsening performance
3% — more of the same
4% — exercise performance cut by 20-30%
5% — headache, irritability, "spaced-out" feeling, fatigue
6% — weakness, severe loss of thermoregulation
7% — collapse is likely unless exercise is stopped

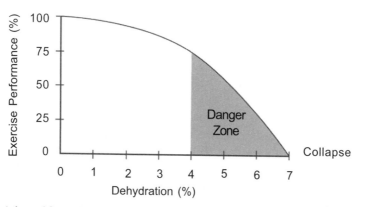

Adapted from Grandjean, A.C. and Ruud, J.S. Nutrition for Cyclists. *Clin Sports Med* 1994;13:235-247.

you would need to consume $3/8$ of a teaspoon of salt with a liter of water every hour. To make sure the salt and water are properly absorbed the beverage also needs to contain 4-8 percent sugar. But the beverage should not be too sweet. Sugar levels above 10 percent are poorly absorbed and can cause diarrhea.

Commercial beverages and sports drinks come up short on the sodium and often have too much sugar. Coconut water is a better option. Although a liter of coconut water may or may not have a full gram of sodium, extra sodium can be added if desired either in the water or separately. In addition, coconut water also replenishes lost trace minerals, has the proper sugar content for optimum absorption, supplies amino acids and other nutrients which may also support proper hydration, and to top it off, it tastes good. All of which makes coconut water an excellent oral rehydration beverage.

"Coconut water improved my performance," says marathon runner Daniel Mondschain. Daniel was introduced to coconut water while training for his fifth marathon. "At first, I drank it only after my runs," says Daniel. "I realized that I was recovering more quickly and with less soreness." Impressed with the results, he began drinking coconut water instead of water or sports beverages during his workouts. He drank only coconut water throughout the final two months of training and during the marathon. The result? "I set a personal record and beat my last time by seven minutes. I had more energy, less fatigue, and less pain in the final miles and that made all the difference." Coconut water is now a permanent fixture in his training regimen.

If you are going to run in an endurance race or participate in some other form of rigorous physical activity, it is wise to prepare yourself beforehand. Just before the activity drink approximately 12-16 ounces (350-500 ml) of water or better yet an electrolyte solution such as coconut water to delay the process of dehydration. Drink frequently while exercising to stay hydrated, 6-12 ounces (150-350 ml) every 15-20 minutes. During training and heat acclimatization, and for several days prior to competition, increase your salt intake to 10-15 grams per day. Sodium is important for recovery so after the event increase your salt intake. This can be done by eating a meal that contains salty foods. Avoid aspirin, ibuprofen and other anti-inflammatories, Tylenol, and antihistamines during exercise and especially during competition.

4

Electrolyte Up
Your Life

THE OCEAN WITHIN US

Water is essential to life. Although we live on dry land, we need a constant source of water every day, at least 3200 ml (13.5 cups). Even our bodies are composed mostly of water, as much as 60 percent. About 90 pounds of the weight of a 150 pound person comes from water. The remaining 60 pounds comprises the solid matter.

Water is found inside and around every living cell in our bodies. It is the solvent in which most other compounds, such as minerals, are dissolved. It is the medium in which most all chemical and electrical reactions in the body take place. The chemical composition of the body's fluids is very precise; it must be because even a slight variation can have serious consequences. Despite influences that constantly affect fluid composition, the body is remarkably effective in responding and maintaining chemical equilibrium.

During the 19th century, scientists were impressed by the similarity between the mineral content of human body fluids and seawater. Influenced by Darwinism, the theory was proposed that all life began from a single-celled organism in the sea. Seawater provided the cells with the nutrients and the chemistry they needed for survival. Over the course of millions of years, multi-celled organisms internalized the ocean—to continue bathing the cells in a warm, mineral rich fluid that keeps them alive. The maintenance of this "internal sea" is so important that it is credited with our ability to live on land. Our body's fluid mineral

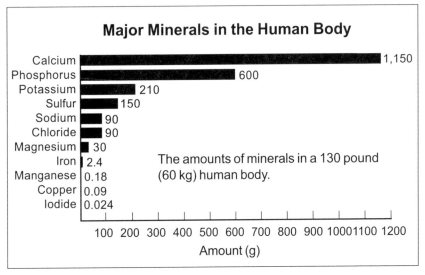

Major Minerals in the Human Body

Mineral	Amount (g)
Calcium	1,150
Phosphorus	600
Potassium	210
Sulfur	150
Sodium	90
Chloride	90
Magnesium	30
Iron	2.4
Manganese	0.18
Copper	0.09
Iodide	0.024

The amounts of minerals in a 130 pound (60 kg) human body.

This graph shows the amounts of the 11 most abundant minerals in the human body. Calcium and phosphorous are the two most abundant minerals. They are found primarily in the bones. The third most abundant mineral is potassium and the fifth and sixth are sodium and chloride, which are found primarily in body fluids. Dozens of other trace minerals are also present but not represented in this graph.

content and temperature are believed to be the same as that of the ocean millions of years ago. The ocean today has become saltier and cooler. But scientists believe we carry the ancient ocean within us.

Whether this theory is accurate or not, it illustrates the fact that the fluids in our bodies contain a large variety of minerals, some in very minute amounts, all of which are necessary for optimal health. Some of these minerals may be toxic in larger quantities but necessary in the proportions they are found in the sea. Major minerals like calcium, sodium, and potassium have a strong influence on our health and we need a relatively large amount. Minor minerals like iodine, zinc, and molybdenum have a less dramatic, but no less essential, impact on our health and our life.

We need the major minerals in relatively large amounts to maintain consistent levels in our body. The loss of even a small percent can have dramatic effects. A drop of just 6 percent in potassium, for instance, can cause complete heart failure. Because the need for trace minerals is much less, a deficiency may be tolerated for a longer period of time. For example, a deficiency in iodine that is not enough to cause severe symptoms yet still is subnormal, can slow down thyroid function. An underactive thyroid may cause low energy, weight gain, irritability, hair loss, depression, dry skin and hair, constipation, reduced resistance to infections, and other symptoms. While these conditions are not in themselves fatal, if the problem is not corrected they can set the stage for more serious health problems later on. A deficiency can exist is any number of trace minerals necessary for optimal health.

The minerals in the sea and in the fluids of our internal sea are in the form of electrolytes. Electrolytes, also known as ions, are atoms or molecules with an electrical charge. Table salt is composed of the elements sodium and chloride. When placed in water the two elements dissolve and split into two separate entities. Each element carries a charge, sodium positive and chloride negative. Because of the charge, they can conduct electricity. If you put wires from both ends of a battery into a glass of salt water an electrical current will flow down one wire across the water and up the other wire. However, if you put the wires in a glass of distilled water, nothing will happen. Since there are no electrolytes in the distilled water, electricity cannot pass. It is because of this electric potential that charged ions are referred to as electrolytes. The ability to carry a charge allows electric current to flow through our bodies and facilitate many biological functions.

In addition to sodium and chloride, there are many other electrolytes. Potassium, calcium, magnesium, phosphate, and sulfate are some of the other major electrolytes. Electrolytes function in many of the essential chemical and electrical reactions that occur in our bodies. Two of the most important and abundant electrolytes in the human body are sodium and potassium. Sodium is the primary electrolyte in the extracellular fluid (outside the cells) and potassium is the primary electrolyte in intracellular fluid (inside the cells).

We get electrolytes from food and drink. We also lose them every day through sweat, urine, etc. So the concentration of electrolytes is continually changing. Our bodies, however, require that we maintain precise amounts of each electrolyte. The kidneys function as our electrolyte controller. If we have too much it filters out the excess and dumps it into the urine for removal. If we need more, it recycles what is present to maintain needed levels. In this way body chemistry is kept in balance.

THE YIN AND YANG OF SODIUM AND POTASSIUM

Everything in nature strives to attain balance or equilibrium with its surroundings. The idea of balance is the basic principle behind traditional oriental medicine. Asians use the concept of yin and yang as a fundamental way of looking at all things, including our bodies and our health.

Yin and yang represent opposites—male and female, hot and cold, wet and dry, and so on. They do not compete, but are complementary, necessary, and inseparable. They coexist and counterbalance each other, just as you cannot have light without darkness, or up without down, you cannot have yin without yang.

In oriental medicine sickness or discomfort arises when there is an imbalance in our bodies—we have too much yin or too much yang. This imbalance creates disharmony and stress and interferes with the natural order of things. Oriental medicine strives to rebalance yin and yang. The physician's job is to assist the patient in rebalancing through therapies that either reduce or increase each one. A simple example is if a patient is dehydrated, say too much yin, the treatment is to give him more fluids, yang. Likewise, the over consumption of water would create the opposite effect and fluids would need to be removed from the body to rebalance. Proper hydration represents a balance in the yin and yang of the body's fluids.

In many ways, sodium and potassium function in a yin-yang relationship—they oppose each other, yet complement each other. Health cannot be maintained without a perfect balance between the two.

Every cell in your body is enclosed by a membrane. This membrane is like a skin that encases the cell's organs and fluids and keeps them separated from surrounding materials. The membrane allows certain substances to enter the cell while blocking the entrance of others. Water, glucose, oxygen, carbon dioxide, and other substances stream in and

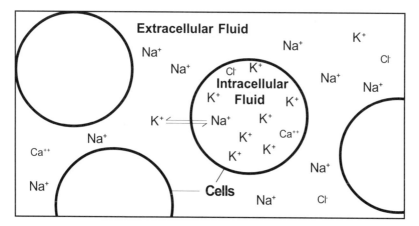

Sodium (Na⁺) concentrates on the outside of cells while potassium (K⁺) is concentrated more on the inside. Sodium and potassium exchange with each other across the cell wall to maintain this balance.

out of the cells in an endless procession. Some substances diffuse easily though the membrane wall, while others require the aid of specialized proteins to shuttle them in or out. The flow of substances in and out of the cells is precisely monitored by electrolytes, principally sodium and potassium.

Potassium is concentrated mostly inside our cells while sodium remains primarily on the outside, although there are some of both in each fluid compartment. This separation of sodium and potassium is important in maintaining fluid volume inside the cell, acid-base balance, and in generating electrical impulses. In short, the difference between the sodium and potassium across the membrane helps the cells do their job. For example, nerve cells use the sodium-potassium distribution across their membranes to generate electricity, making it possible for nerve impulses to travel and for muscles to contract—allowing us to think and to move. This is why dehydration and electrolyte depletion during exercise can severely affect physical performance and endurance.

During nerve transmission and muscle contraction, potassium and sodium briefly exchange places across the cell membrane. The cell then quickly pumps them back into place. This makes sodium and potassium critical in the transmission of messages along nerves and from nerves to muscles, as well as in the response of muscles, including the heart muscle, to those messages.

The kidneys aid in maintaining sodium-potassium balance. When sodium intake is low, for example, potassium excretion is higher. In this way the body's sodium and potassium levels remain in balance.

OUR BODY'S NEED FOR SODIUM

Sodium is an essential nutrient. You need it to be healthy. The primary source of sodium in the diet is from sodium chloride—salt. Sodium is found naturally in most foods to some degree or another. Adding salt to foods also increases our dietary intake. Because we normally get adequate amounts of sodium in our diet, little attention is given to sodium deficiency. However despite the abundance of sodium in the diet, sodium deficiency is an often ignored but widespread problem, as we have seen in previous chapters.

We need a steady and consist source of sodium in our diet. As you've seen above, with potassium it is involved in many important physiological functions that keep us alive.

The ability of the kidneys to regulate the sodium and water content of the body is remarkable. Sodium is absorbed easily from the intestinal tract; it then travels in the blood, where it ultimately passes through the kidneys. The kidneys filter all the sodium out, and then with great precision returns to the bloodstream the exact amount of sodium needed. Normally, the amount excreted equals the amount ingested that day.

The blood concentration of sodium rises after a person eats salty foods or meals high in carbohydrate. Carbohydrate also causes sodium retention, an effect of insulin and glucose on the kidney's regulatory mechanisms. Conversely starvation and low carbohydrate diets increase sodium excretion. The high blood concentration stimulates thirst receptors in the brain, and the person drinks until the sodium-to-water ratio reaches a target level. Then the kidneys excrete the extra water together with the extra sodium.

The adult human body contains on average about 100 grams of sodium. Of this, some 30 to 40 percent is located in the bones. A small amount, about 10 percent, gets inside of the cells, but about 60 percent or so is located in extracellular fluids.

Our foods usually contain more sodium than the body needs. Therefore, a minimum Recommended Dietary Allowance (RDA) for sodium has not been set. However the US National Research Council, which sets the RDAs, has estimated the minimum requirement as 500 mg per day. The American Heart Association recommends limiting sodium intake to less than 3 grams daily.* To put these figures in perspective as they relate to salt consumption, that would equate to a minimum requirement of 1.25 grams salt (1/5 teaspoon) and a maximum of 7.5 grams salt (1.25 teaspoons).

The average sodium consumption in the US is estimated to be 4 to 6 grams daily (equivalent to 10 to 15 grams of salt, or 1.67 to 2.5 teaspoons). For most people this amount is adequate to prevent deficiency under most circumstances, but in a small group of sodium sensitive individuals this may be too much and may lead to elevated blood pressure. Sodium sensitivity is defined as an increase in blood pressure in response to a higher sodium chloride intake than that in the baseline diet. It is estimated that in those people who have high blood pressure, about 10 percent are sodium sensitive and can benefit from limiting salt consumption. This amounts to about 2.5 percent of the population. The rest of us can easily handle sodium intake at current levels.[1]

At one time excess sodium or salt consumption was blamed for many people's high blood pressure. But research has shown this is not the case. Treating high blood pressure with salt restricted diets, for the most part, has proven to be unsuccessful. Sodium concentration in the blood and other body tissues is maintained by the kidneys, the adrenal glands, the pituitary gland, and other glands. Most people can, therefore, safely consume more sodium than they need, and rely on these control mechanisms to regulate its excretion and retention as needed.[2] While sodium may exert only a minor influence in blood pressure in most people, the 2.5 percent of the population who are salt sensitive may

---

*Many countries set their own limits on nutritional needs. In the UK the maximum for sodium is set at 1.6 grams per day.

need to restrict their sodium intake. People with chronic kidney disease, those who have parents with hypertension, blacks, and persons over 50 years of age are the most likely to be sodium or salt sensitive.[3]

THE MIRACLE OF POTASSIUM

Potassium is one of the most important minerals in the human body and absolutely essential for good health and life itself. Our bodies contain more than twice as much potassium as they do sodium. A 130 pound (60 kg) person has about 210 grams of potassium and 90 grams of sodium. Ninety-eight percent of the potassium in our bodies is inside our cells. It is the principal electrolyte in our cells.

Besides working in concert with sodium to maintain water balance and controlling nerve and muscle function, potassium has many additional duties. Potassium is involved in the conversion of blood sugar into glycogen for storage in the liver and muscles. Inadequate glycogen storage leads to physical and mental fatigue. It stimulates insulin production. Evidence is showing that it is involved in bone calcification and in maintaining joint health. Potassium buffers acids in the body helping to maintain alkalinity of body fluids. Potassium is a cofactor in many reactions, especially those involving energy production and muscle synthesis. It is especially needed when tissue is being formed, as in growing children or muscle building. During the oxidation of carbohydrates and fats into energy, a number of enzymes are involved—all of which depend on potassium for their stability.

Potassium is found inside of all living cells in both plants and animals. Many of the richest sources of potassium are fresh foods, especially fruits, vegetables, and legumes. Since potassium is available from a variety of foods, no RDA has been established. However, 3500 mg a day is the most commonly cited estimate for a safe and an adequate amount. The US Department of Health and Human Services suggests a daily intake of 4700 mg.

Despite its great importance, potassium is an often overlooked nutrient. Nutritionists haven't given it much attention because it is found in so many foods that unless there are clear signs of malnutrition, a deficiency is believed to be unlikely. Recent research, however, is finding that potassium deficiency is far more common than previously expected.

Many health care professionals believe it may be one of the keys to fighting the increasing incidence of degenerative diseases that plague our society today.

Several studies have indicated that a potassium deficiency exists in as many as 20 percent of all hospitalized patients.[4] In addition, about 14 percent of those people who visit the doctor for various complaints have low potassium levels.

Symptoms of low potassium can vary from mild to severe depending on the severity and duration of the deficiency. Symptoms include:

Muscle weakness
Tiredness or low energy
Muscle cramps
Tingling or numbness
Slow reflexes
Paralysis
Nausea or vomiting
Abdominal cramping, bloating
Constipation and digestive problems
Arrhythmia (irregular heart beat)
Neurological problems (depression, confusion, mental fatigue)
Feelings of malaise

As researchers investigate the role potassium has on our health they are discovering associations between low potassium and many common health problems, particularly in relation to cardiovascular health. The following sections discuss some of the conditions affected by potassium.

Blood Pressure

Hypertension (high blood pressure) affects approximately 25 percent of the adult population worldwide, and its prevalence is predicted to increase by 60 percent over the next 20 years. It is the major risk factor for cardiovascular disease which is responsible for most deaths worldwide.[5]

In the United States high blood pressure contributes to half a million strokes and over a million heart attacks each year. The higher the blood pressure is above normal, the greater the risk. Low blood pressure is believed to be a sign of low risk for heart disease.

The relationship between dietary potassium and blood pressure has been recognized at least since the 1920s.[6] Medical investigators believe potassium might both prevent and treat hypertension. Evidence shows that a high potassium intake protects against stroke and a low intake raises blood pressure.[7]

A number of studies have shown the effectiveness of increasing dietary potassium in controlling high blood pressure. Researchers at the University of Naples in Italy took 54 patients who were on antihypertensive drug therapy. Over a one year period they increased the amount of potassium-rich foods in their diets. At the end of the study period 55 percent reported a significant reduction in symptoms related to their hypertension and 38 percent had completely discontinued medication altogether.[8]

Vegetarians, by the nature of their diets, generally consume a higher amount of potassium than non-vegetarians and typically have lower blood pressure. To test the hypothesis that high fruit and vegetable consumption affects blood pressure, researchers at Johns Hopkins Medical School took 459 individuals with moderately high blood pressure and fed them a controlled diet for eight weeks. The high fruit and vegetable diet produced a noticeable reduction in blood pressure within just two weeks, which was maintained throughout the testing period. Potassium intake amounted to 4.4 grams a day. The researchers concluded that a high potassium diet could serve as an effective alternative to drug therapy in people with moderately high blood pressure.[9]

A question one might ask: is it the potassium in the diet or some other nutrient or combination of nutrients that exerts this blood pressure lowering effect? A group of seven medical researchers from Johns Hopkins University reviewed 33 published studies involving over 2600 participants taking potassium supplements. They concluded that potassium supplementation is effective in lowering blood pressure. People with elevated blood pressure show the most dramatic decrease, but even those with normal blood pressure show a slight decrease as well. While other nutrients may help, it appears that potassium is a key component. Since lower blood pressure is believed to protect against conditions that lead to heart attacks and strokes, a reduction reduces the risk even when values are within a range that are considered normal. Again the researchers recommended the use of potassium as a means to prevent and treat high blood pressure.[10] Studies have shown that simply lowering sodium (salt) consumption has little effect on reducing high blood pressure. Low potassium consumption appears to be far more significant and may be the major factor in the development of high blood pressure. Eating the recommended 5 to 7 servings of fruits and vegetables a day is one way to help prevent hypertension.

Atherosclerosis and Heart Disease

One of the consequences of high blood pressure is the development of atherosclerosis—hardening of the arteries. High blood pressure causes excessive stress within the artery walls, which creates minute tears along the inside of the artery. As with any injury, inflammation results. If blood pressure remains elevated, stress on the artery wall continues and inflammation becomes chronic. Chronic inflammation causes the build up of scar tissue and the deposition of fat, protein, and calcium, forming plaque. Plaque clogs arteries, thus blocking the flow of blood and the delivery of oxygen and nutrients to tissues and organs. Blocking the flow of blood to the heart causes a heart attack; blocking the flow to the brain results in a stroke.

In populations where the consumption of potassium is high, cardiovascular disease is low. High fruit and vegetable consumption in modern diets is also associated with a reduced risk of heart disease. In studies in humans and in animals there is a strong association between low potassium intake and hypertension, stroke, and other cardiovascular conditions.

Potassium is a heart protective nutrient. As noted previously a deficiency in potassium can cause an abnormal heartbeat (arrhythmia) which can weaken and disrupt proper heart function. And in cases of severe deficiency it can cause the heart to stop beating altogether. As you've just seen above, it also helps reduce high blood pressure—a major risk factor for heart disease. Potassium also appears to protect the lining within the artery wall from developing plaque, which is the underlying cause of heart disease.

Potassium protects against atherosclerosis in other ways. It has been shown to inhibit free-radical formation in arterial tissues, reduce platelet aggregation, and reduce the formation of blood clots. In special diets designed to promote atherosclerosis in lab animals, reducing the potassium content increases atherosclerotic lesions and increasing potassium reduces lesions, thus demonstrating a clear association between potassium intake and risk of developing atherosclerosis.[11-12]

Potassium has a remarkable ability to protect the heart even when the organ is subjected to a variety of toxins that can cause a fatal heart attack. Dr. P. Prioreschi reviewed 13 studies in which a variety of potentially fatal poisons, which target and seriously damage the heart, were essentially nullified by the administration of potassium. "It is quite obvious," states Prioreschi, "that potassium shows an astonishing capacity to protect the myocardium (heart) against a wide variety of cardiotoxic agents." Since potassium can protect the heart even after it has been subjected to heart damaging agents, Prioreschi suggests that it may be useful in the prevention of heart attacks as well.[13]

Stroke

Numerous studies have found an association between low potassium consumption and increased risk of stroke.[14-17] Research has shown that those people who eat the highest amount of potassium-rich fruits and vegetables have a significantly reduced chance of suffering a stroke. The same degree of protection can also be obtained from taking potassium supplements.

"Other components of fruits and vegetables may also contribute to the reduced risk of stroke, but this beneficial effect appears to be due to the high potassium content of these diets," says Alberto Ascherio, MD, associate professor of nutrition and epidemiology at Harvard School of Public Health. Ascherio headed one of the largest studies to date on the relationship between potassium and stroke. His study included almost 44,000 men between the ages of 40 and 75 years. None of which had diagnosed cardiovascular disease or diabetes. Over an eight year period 328 strokes were reported. Researchers found that individuals in the top fifth of dietary potassium intake (mean intake 4.3 g/d) had a 38 percent lower risk of stroke than those in the bottom fifth (mean intake 2.4 g/d). The major difference between the diets of the two groups was in their consumption of fruits and vegetables—about nine servings daily in the highest potassium group compared with four in the lowest. Those who used potassium supplements also demonstrated lower risk.[18] Individuals who had high blood pressure (8520) and were taking potassium supplements (about 1 gram a day) had a 60 percent reduced risk of stroke when compared to those with high blood pressure who weren't taking supplements.

Although some of the protective effect provided by potassium was due to the lowering of blood pressure, Ascherio says the decrease in stroke did not appear to be due solely to changes in blood pressures. There are other factors such as dilation of blood vessels, reducing platelet stickiness, and reducing blood clot formation which also contribute to potassium's protective effects.

The research findings on the reduced risk of stroke and high blood pressure associated with potassium are so strong that the US National Academy of Science (NAS) states in their official report *Diet and Health: Implications for Reducing Chronic Disease Risk*, "Epidemiological and animal studies indicate that the risk of stroke-related deaths is inversely related to potassium intake over the entire range of blood pressures, and the relationship appears to be dose dependent. The combination of a low-sodium, high potassium intake is associated with the lowest blood pressure levels and the lowest frequency of stroke in individuals and populations. Although the effects of reducing sodium intake and increasing potassium intake would vary and may be small in some individuals, the estimated reduction in stroke-related mortality for the population is large." This statement is endorsed by FDA.

Bone and Joint Health

Bone size and density increases in early life and peaks around the age of 20. At about the age of 30 or 40 we start to lose bone mass. We continue to lose bone mass throughout the rest of our lives. Because women's bones are less dense than men's and their hormonal changes accelerate losses, osteoporosis is eight times more common in women than in men.

While bone loss is a natural process that cannot be completely prevented, it can be minimized. Those who are most susceptible to developing osteoporosis are those who do not reach their full physical potential in their younger years. The amount and quality of the bone laid down in those early years and maintained throughout midlife depends primarily on the diet. If we eat a well-balanced diet while young, to build dense bones, and continue to eat well throughout adulthood bone loss is minimized.

Calcium is the primary building block of the skeleton and adequate dietary intake is essential for building strong bones. Vitamins A and D as well as phosphorus, magnesium, silicon, and boron are also needed. Potassium, too, is essential, especially later in life because it helps prevent bone loss.

Excessive excretion of calcium as we age reduces the amount of this mineral in the body, meaning there is less available to be utilized in bone formation and maintenance. Studies show that when potassium consumption is low, calcium excretion increases.[19]

Potassium and calcium are alkalizing elements. Diets high in acid forming foods (meats and grains) acidify the body. Heavy exercise also increases acidity. Calcium is used to buffer the acid, and in the process, is pulled out of the body. Potassium can also buffer the acid and thereby, reduce the amount of calcium used up in this process.[20]

What happens to the calcium that remains in the body? It is used, among other things, to maintain bone health. Potassium apparently is particularly effective in neutralizing excess acid. It is even better than magnesium, another alkalizing element. Studies show that potassium supplementation or diets high in potassium-rich foods increase bone mineral density.[21-22]

We are often counseled to get plenty of calcium in our diets and are encouraged to drink milk and eat dairy products because they are rich sources of this nutrient. Yet, despite eating lots of dairy and taking calcium supplements, osteoporosis remains a serious problem for older people. Eating too much calcium has drawbacks, such as developing kidney stones. And higher calcium consumption doesn't always equate to stronger bones. Other nutrients are also required. Focusing on just one nutrient won't solve the problem. This may explain why women in many underdeveloped countries who have a low calcium (i.e., dairy) intake, even less then the US RDA, have excellent bone health even into old age.

If you want to build strong bones while you are young and want to maintain them as you age, eating a potassium-rich diet, which also supplies calcium and other essential nutrients, is a smart move.

Healthy bones and healthy joints go together. Arthritis is a process in which joints degenerate. Arthritis sufferers have been found to have low potassium levels.[23] This suggests that potassium may also help to keep joints strong and healthy and ward off degenerative joint disease. That's the belief of Dr. Reza Rastmanesh. He performed a large controlled clinical trial testing potassium supplements against rheumatoid arthritis and reported dramatic decreases in pain in all the patients.

Heat Stroke and Exercise Performance

Several studies suggest that potassium depletion may play an important role in the development of heat exhaustion and affect exercise performance. Studies indicate that those people who suffer from heat cramps, heat exhaustion, and heat stroke during hot weather have low levels of potassium.[24]

Low potassium levels also affect muscle strength and exercise performance. In one study, for instance, rats were split into two groups. The diet given to each group was identical except for the potassium content. The potassium in one group was 16 times greater than the other. When the animals were run until exhaustion, the low potassium fed rats accomplished only half of the work done by the high potassium group. The low potassium group also exhibited much greater heat gain, making them more susceptible to heat exhaustion.[25]

During heavy exercise the main source of energy comes from glycogen (glucose stored in muscle tissue). This results in the production of a high amount of lactic acid in the muscles. The soreness you feel in your muscles after a hard workout is due primarily from lactic acid buildup. The buildup of lactic acid is believed to contribute to muscular fatigue by reducing muscle and blood pH levels, a state called metabolic acidosis.

It is believed that preventing this state of acidosis may improve exercise performance and buffering agents have been recommended to accomplish this.[26] Sodium citrate and sodium bicarbonate supplements are the most common buffering agents used. The problem with these is that it takes about 1-3 hours after ingestion for them to have an effect and they often cause ingestion. Another possible solution is to eat a high potassium diet. Potassium will also alkalize excess acids in the blood, thus helping to reduce lactic acid buildup and optimize exercise performance.

Digestive Health
Potassium is well absorbed from foods in the digestive tract. Muscles, including those along the digestive tract, require potassium to function properly. Without adequate potassium muscle function declines. The muscles that line our digestive tract push digesting foods through the stomach, small intestine, and large intestine (colon). If these muscles become weakened they cannot perform this function in an efficient manner. The consequence? Constipation and other digestive problems such as heartburn, hemorrhoids, diverticulitis, and perhaps irritable bowel syndrome and cancer. Studies have shown that a serious potassium deficiency in animals leads to such severe constipation that animals may die.

When we suffer from poor digestion, constipation, and related problems the cause may be related to low potassium. In fact, a lack of potassium is often found in people who have digestive complaints, including Crohn's disease.[27]

A natural health remedy for constipation is potassium and prunes. Besides aiding in muscular contractions, potassium is reported to draw water out of the colon and into the fecal matter, thus making it softer and easier to move along the colon and be eliminated. An anti-constipation beverage can be made by combining prunes with coconut water. Start by soaking a few prunes in a glass of hot water for about 10 minutes to soften. Drain water and allow prunes to cool. Put the softened prunes and coconut water in a blender and blend together. Drink the beverage on an empty stomach in the morning.

PUT POTASSIUM INTO YOUR DIET
Is Your Yin Out of Balance with Your Yang?
Potassium is well absorbed from foods, but is not stored in significantly large amounts in the body, so we need to consume it daily

to satisfy the body's needs. Most natural foods—fruits, vegetables, legumes, and meats contain ample amounts of potassium. Processed and packaged foods, baked goods, canned fruits and vegetables, heat-and-serve meals, ready-to-eat cereals, and luncheon meats are depleted in potassium and enriched with sodium. Most of the foods people eat nowadays are highly processed and, therefore, potassium poor and sodium rich. This is just the opposite of what the diet consisted of a couple of generations ago and throughout history, before the advent of modern food processing. Currently we consume about three and a half times more sodium than we do potassium.

Isolated populations that continue to eat the same foods as they have eaten for generations eat three to ten times more potassium as they do sodium, just the opposite of what we typically eat.[28-30] Hypertension affects less than 1 percent of people in isolated societies but almost one third of adults in industrialized countries. When people in isolated societies move into urban areas, blood pressure and incidence of stroke increases, reflecting their change in diet.[31-32] A decrease in potassium consumption is one of those changes.

Our kidneys are designed to conserve sodium and excrete potassium. Prehistoric humans, who consumed a sodium-poor and potassium-rich diet, were well suited to this mechanism. With such a diet, sodium excretion is negligible and potassium excretion is high, matching potassium intake. This mechanism, however, is turned upside down with our modern sodium-rich and potassium-poor diet. The end result is the failure of the kidneys to adapt and the increased risk of developing hypertension and related conditions.

Since our bodies contain more than twice as much potassium as sodium, it is logical to assume that a healthy diet should also contain at least twice as much potassium as sodium. Some authorities believe a 4:1 ratio is better. The tables on pages 76 and 77 list the potassium and sodium content of various foods. Notice that the potassium content of most fresh foods is typically 5, 10, 20 or more times higher than sodium. These are the types of foods humans have been eating for generations, at a time before heart disease became a worldwide crisis. However, in processed foods sodium content is significantly higher than potassium.

Many people are subclinically potassium deficient, in other words, they consume just enough potassium to prevent outward deficiency

SODIUM AND POTASSIUM CONTENT IN FOODS

Food	Quantity/Size	Sodium (mg)	Potassium (mg)
Apple	1 medium	1	148
Apple Cider Vinegar	1 cup	12	174
Asparagus, cooked	1 cup	26	404
Avocado	1	11	690
Banana	1 medium	1	422
Blackberries	1 cup	1	233
Blueberries	1 cup	1	114
Broccoli	1 cup chopped	30	288
Carrot	1 medium	42	195
Cantaloupe	1 cup, diced	25	417
Cauliflower, raw	1 cup	30	303
Celery, raw	1 cup	81	263
Cherries	1 cup without pits	0	322
Coconut Water (inland)*	1 cup	27	451
Coconut Water (shoreline)*	1 cup	252	600
Grapes, seedless	1 cup	3	288
Green Beans, cooked	1 cup	1	215
Green Peppers, raw	1 cup c hopped	4	261
Kelp, raw	1 cup	184	72
Kidney Beans, cooked	1 cup	9	669
Lettuce, green leaf,	1 cup, shredded	10	70
Lima Beans, cooked	1 cup	5	730
Mango	1 cup	3	257
Oatmeal, cooked	1 cup	2	131
Onion, raw	1 cup	6	234
Papaya	1 cup	4	360
Peaches	1 cup	0	293
Peas, cooked	1 cup	5	434
Pear	1 cup	2	192
Pineapple	1 cup	2	178
Potato, cooked	1 medium	8	610
Raspberries	1 cup	1	186
Rice, brown cooked	1 cup	10	162
Rice, white cooked	1 cup	2	55
Spinach, raw	1 cup	24	167
Strawberries	1 cup	2	254
Tomato, raw	1 cup, chopped	9	427
Watermelon	1 cup	2	170

SODIUM AND POTASSIUM CONTENT IN PREPARED FOODS

Food	Quantity/Size	Sodium (mg)	Potassium (mg)
Angel Food Cake	1 piece	254	68
Bagel, plain enriched	1 medium	255	43
Bacon, cooked	1 slice	185	45
Bologna, beef	1 slice	302	48
Beef Stew	1 cup	984	396
Brotwurst	1 link	778	197
Cheese Crackers	1 cup	617	90
Chicken Noodle Soup	1 cup	850	108
Chocolate Chip Cookies	2 large	119	59
Cola	1 cup	7	3
Corn Chex	1 cup	280	45
Corn Chips	3 ounces	523	114
Cottage Cheese, low fat	1 cup	918	194
Donut	1 medium	232	60
Enchilada, cheese	1	784	240
Froot Loops	1 cup	150	36
Hamburger	1	551	220
Ham, lunch meat	1 slice	365	80
Lasagna	4 ounces	324	208
Lucky Charms	1 cup	200	50
Onion Rings	8-9 rings	430	129
Popsicle	1	6	6
Pretzels	10 twist	814	82
Rice Krispies	1 cup	266	31
Salami	1 slice	296	49
Sprite	1 cup	22	2
Taco, beef	1	349	168
Toaster Pastry	1	181	41
Wheat Bread	1 slice	130	46
White Bread	1 slice	170	25

*Due to their access to seawater, coconuts grown near the seashore contain a higher percentage of sodium than those grown inland.

Source: USDA National Nutrient Database for Standard Reference (2006) and Eiseman, B. Intravenous infusion of coconut water. *A.M.A. Archives of Surgerey* 1954;68:167-178.

symptoms but they are still lacking this essential nutrient. They are walking the edge of potassium deficiency. A slight disruption in potassium levels could easily throw them over the edge. Extreme dieting or semi-fasts, illness (especially if it involves vomiting or diarrhea), heavy exercise or sweating, and medications (diuretics, laxatives, and hormone products) can all deplete already low levels of potassium. As in the case of heavy exercise or illness, potassium levels can drop to dangerously low levels in a relatively short amount of time. If the diet is lacking in fresh fruits and vegetables, depletion occurs more quickly. Consequently, potassium deficiency is becoming a more common, yet still under diagnosed problem.

When sodium consumption is high, the need for potassium also increases to help maintain electrolyte balance; remember the concept of yin and yang? Unfortunately, our diets are high in sodium and low in potassium. The fact that some populations have very high salt intakes, yet have low rates of heart attacks and strokes, gives credence to the idea that health is more of a food balance issue than it is an excess or deficiency of any one particular nutrient. Since our diet is typically high in sodium and low in potassium, it appears evident that we need to add more potassium rich foods into our diet to maintain balance.

The International Study of Salt and Blood Pressure (INTERSALT) which included 10,079 subjects from 32 countries, showed an average consumption of 9.9 g of salt a day. Experimental studies show that most people tolerate a wide range of sodium intakes, from about 250 mg to 30,000 mg a day.[33] Some people are more sensitive to the effects of sodium than others. People who are sodium sensitive retain sodium more easily, leading to excess fluid retention and increased blood pressure. If you are in that group, excess sodium in your diet increases your chance of developing high blood pressure. A healthy person can tolerate a much higher upper limit.

Where salt is readily available the vast majority of the world's population chooses to consume 6 to 10 grams of salt per day. In certain populations in Japan, where salty foods are popular, salt consumption can average an incredible 26 grams or more a day.[34] The national average in Japan is 11.4 grams a day. Despite the high salt diet, the Japanese have one of the highest life expectancies in the world and a relatively low rate of heart disease.

How can some people eat large quantities of sodium and still not develop high blood pressure? Recent studies show that high sodium intake alone does not cause high blood pressure.[35] Researchers now recognize that it is neither an excess in sodium, nor a deficiency in potassium alone that promotes high blood pressure, but an imbalance between sodium and potassium. This explains why some populations can have a high sodium diet but normal blood pressure, because potassium consumption is also high. This has been demonstrated in lab animals. Increasing the potassium intake of hypertensive rats that were fed high sodium diets lowers blood pressure, reduces the incidence of stroke and stroke-related death, and prevents cardiac hypertrophy, mesenteric vascular damage, and renal injury.[36]

What about the 2.5 percent of people who are sodium sensitive? Dietary potassium has been shown to exert a powerful, dose-dependent inhibitory effect on sodium sensitivity. In fact, studies show that an increase in dietary potassium can even "abolish" sodium sensitivity in hypertensive subjects.[37]

A Coconut A Day Keeps Strokes Away

"Potassium depletion as a risk factor for stroke: will a banana a day keep your stroke away?" This was the title of an article that appeared in the November 2002 issue of the medical journal *Neurology*. In 2002 the United States Food and Drug Administration (FDA) gave approval to the banana industry allowing them to make a health claim on their products stating that eating bananas can reduce risk of stroke and high blood pressure.

When we think of sources of potassium most of us automatically think of bananas. Bananas have long been regarded as a good source of potassium, and they are—a medium size banana contains about 422 mg of potassium. Although bananas are often mentioned as an excellent way to get potassium, they are not the only source, nor the richest source. One of the highest sources of potassium is coconut water. One cup of coconut water supplies 600 mg of potassium—more than a banana. Most fresh coconuts and commercially bottled coconut water contain about 12 ounces of fluid or approximately 900 mg of potassium per serving. That beats bananas hands down.

How does this compare with other sources of potassium? You would have to eat nearly six cups of shredded cabbage to equal the amount of potassium you get in one cup of coconut water. You would need to eat five large grapefruits, or 12 cups of white rice, or eight cups of raw kelp to get the same amount. Apple cider vinegar is often touted as a health tonic and does have many benefits. Experts have claimed that much of, if not most of, the health benefits ascribed to apple cider vinegar are due to its high potassium content. As far as potassium goes, it can't compare to coconut water. You would need to drink a full *quart* of apple cider vinegar to get the same amount of potassium you would from a singe cup of coconut water—and drinking the coconut water would be far more enjoyable!

The FDA states that potassium-rich foods that meet its standards may carry language on their packaging that carries the claim: "Diets containing foods that are good sources of potassium and low in sodium may reduce the risk of high blood pressure and stroke."

To qualify to use this statement a product must be a good source of potassium (contain 10 percent or more of the Daily Value for potassium) and be low in sodium. Therefore, qualifying foods must have at least 350 mg of potassium per serving and 140 mg or less of sodium. In addition, qualifying foods also must be low in fat, low in saturated fat, and low in cholesterol. A serving is typically regarded as half a cup. Coconut water easily fits these criteria. Therefore, here is an endorsement from the FDA. Studies do show that coconut water can be used to control high blood pressure.[38] Since coconut water is a richer source of potassium than bananas you can say: "a coconut a day keeps strokes away."

How to Get More Potassium into Your Diet?

The average American diet supplies between 1500 to 5000 mg of potassium a day. Most Western countries probably have a similar intake. The US Department of Health and Human Services recommends that we get 4600 mg a day. Therefore, the vast majority of people are consuming suboptimal amounts of potassium.

In contrast, the average consumption of sodium is between 4000 and 6000 mg a day. Therefore, most people are consuming almost twice as much sodium as they are potassium. This is the exact opposite

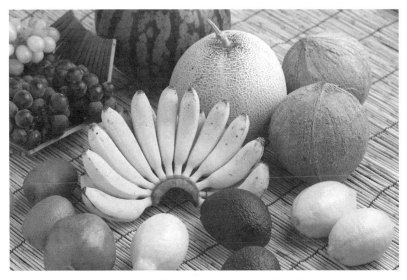

The FDA allows food producers to make health claims on the consumption of certain fruits and vegetables.

of what is believed to be desirable. Seventy-seven percent of the sodium in our foods comes from eating prepared or processed food with added salt; 12 percent is from natural sources and 11 percent is added during cooking or while eating.

Simply cutting down on processed or packaged foods would dramatically reduce sodium consumption and help to balance sodium-potassium intake. It is recommended that we get at least 5 servings and as much as 9 servings a day of fruits and vegetables. Most people don't get the minimum 5 servings. Eating fresh fruits and vegetables not only supplies many nutrients, besides potassium, but reduces sodium consumption and displaces less nutritious foods that would otherwise be eaten.

Twelve ounces of coconut water, the amount in one coconut, contains about 900 mg of potassium. Coconut water counts as part of the daily fruit and vegetable recommendation. Drinking the water from five coconuts will supply more than enough to meet the US Department of Health's recommendations. You certainly don't need to drink that many daily, but one or two a day can go a long way in fulfilling your potassium requirement.

Since coconut water is such a good source of potassium, some people might worry that they may get too much from their diet and from drinking coconut water. Getting too much potassium is not a problem. Our bodies can tolerate a very high amount of potassium. We cannot get too much potassium from eating foods. We can safely consume far more potassium than we need. Our bodies simply eliminate the excess. The only way to get too much potassium is by taking potassium supplements or medications and then the body responds by vomiting to expel the excess.

Coconut water is an excellent source of potassium, but it is not an excessive source, nor the most abundant food source. There are other foods with higher potassium levels. So don't think that drinking three or four glasses of coconut water a day is going to give you toxic levels of potassium. You couldn't drink enough in a day to overdose on potassium. The only precaution with large amounts of potassium may be with people who have serious kidney disease and are incapable of filtering out large quantities of minerals.

Besides potassium, coconut water also provides many other essential electrolytes. Drinking one or more glasses of coconut water daily can be one of the healthiest things you can do.

MINERALS FROM THE SEA

Coconuts grow in tropical climates near the seashore where they have access to both fresh and salt water. Seawater with its high mineral content acts as sort of a fertilizer to coconut palms. The trees grow faster and produce better when they have access to a certain amount of seawater. Although coconut palms can grow many miles inland, they do better if seawater is available.

Seawater is a rich source of minerals. In fact, seawater contains a complete mixture of all major and trace minerals. There are about 65 different minerals in nature and all of them are found to some extent in seawater.

These minerals, which apparently aid the coconut in its growth and development, are absorbed into the roots and, by way of the sap, delivered throughout the tree and into the fruit—the coconut. Consequently, coconut water contains a variety of minerals from the

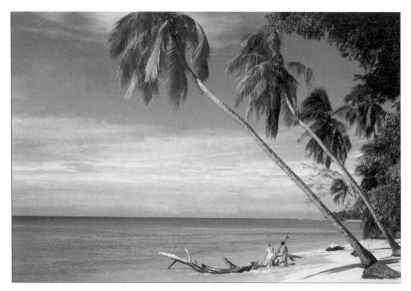

The ocean is an abundent source of minerals.

sea. Coconut water contains the major minerals such as sodium, magnesium, potassium, as well as the minor minerals zinc, selenium, iron, manganese, boron, copper, sulfur, iodine, molybdenum, and others.[39] Trace minerals are present in very small amounts just as they are in seawater.

A solution of water and dissolved minerals (salts) makes up the "internal sea" of the body. Our bodies need the different minerals to make tissues, enzymes, and hormones. Even trace minerals, which by definition come in very small or "trace" amounts, are important to overall health.

Ordinary water, even mineral rich water, is not a good source of minerals. These minerals are derived from rock and are difficult for the body to absorb and utilize. Plants can take inorganic minerals and convert them into compounds that make them more useable by our bodies.

Therefore, fruits, vegetables, and other foods are our primary source of minerals. One of the shortcomings of modern food production is the lack of trace minerals. Soils that have been repeatedly farmed for many years are seriously depleted of trace minerals. Consequently, the foods grown on these farms are also deficient. Foods from the sea, however, are good sources of trace minerals because they have access to mineral-rich seawater. Likewise, coconut water can provide trace minerals. The minerals in coconut water are in an easily absorbable ionic form. The indigenous populations of the Pacific islands are generally aware of the "saltier" taste of coconut water obtained from coconuts growing near the ocean.[40] The trace mineral content may be another reason why coconut water works so well as an intravenous and oral rehydration fluid.

5

A Health Tonic

COCONUT WATER'S BALANCING ACT

Have you ever seen a group of acrobats or cheerleaders form a human pyramid? Each member of the group is carefully positioned within the pyramid with an assigned job of holding onto or balancing on top of other members. Each member is connected to two, three, or more of the others. If just one member of the group is not properly balanced or slips, the entire pyramid comes tumbling down.

Our bodies also perform a delicate balancing act. Doctors call this homeostasis. Homeostasis is dynamic, that is, it is constantly adjusting to environmental influences to maintain internal equilibrium, just as acrobats constantly shift their weight to maintain balance. Homeostasis plays a vital role in maintaining health because tissues and organs can function efficiently only within a narrow range of conditions. Factors that affect homeostasis include blood pH, water content, electrolyte levels, blood sugar levels, hormone levels, temperature, among others.

Our bodies perform their best when they maintain a temperature of 98.6 degrees F. Raising or lowering the temperature just a few degrees can bring on unpleasant symptoms. A shift of temperature of just 10 degrees for an extended period of time can have serious and even fatal consequences. Likewise, blood pH needs to be maintained at a very narrow range of 7.35-7.45. Outside this range, if correction isn't made quickly, it brings on sickness. If pH extends past a range of 6.8-8.0, death follows.

Whenever there is an imbalance, the body is quick to try to correct it. If an imbalance lasts too long or becomes chronic, symptoms of disease may arise: fatigue, aches, pains, vision disturbances, heartburn, constipation, arthritis, osteoporosis, hypoglycemia, and such are all the result of the body being out of balance.

Coconut water appears to have an amazing ability to help the body maintain homeostasis, particularly in regards to fluid and electrolyte balance. As we have seen in previous chapters, coconut water is an excellent rehydration fluid. It also helps balance pH and electrolyte levels.

One of the unique features about coconut water is its *biodirectional* character. Unlike a drug that pushes the body in one direction or another, coconut water can move the body in the direction it needs to go. If the body is dehydrated, it can rehydrate it. If the body is over hydrated, it can cause the removal of excess water. Whether coconut water is pulling excess fluid out or replenishing depleted fluids, electrolyte and pH balance is maintained.

Previously, the biggest concern doctors had about using coconut water as a rehydration medium was its electrolyte profile. Its relatively high potassium and low sodium content gives it a diuretic effect when the body is well hydrated. However, coconut water is an excellent rehydration fluid for those people who are dehydrated. Despite its high potassium level, mineral imbalances don't occur because any excess is excreted in the urine and other minerals, such as sodium, are recycled.

Coconut water has long been known as a natural diuretic. Diuretics are substances that promote or stimulate the production of urine. Diuretics are among the most commonly used drugs in medicine. They are useful because they influence water and electrolyte balance, especially sodium and potassium. Some of the most common conditions for which diuretics are used include: edema (water retention), hypertension (high blood pressure), congestive heart failure, kidney disease, liver disease (cirrhosis), glaucoma, and hyponatermia (low blood sodium).

Coconut water is not like most diuretic drugs. Drugs affect electrolyte balance and hormones to force water removal. Coconut water, as well as many other diuretic-like herbs, is classified as an aquaretic. Aquaretics, in contrast to diuretics, are kidney-friendly herbs that stimulate urine production without affecting hormones or electrolyte levels. Only water is affected. Pharmaceutical companies are now actively developing aquaretic drugs because they do not have the drawbacks associated with conventional diuretics. One of the major drawbacks to some of the diuretic drugs is that they pull potassium out of the body and promote hypokalemia (low blood potassium). Coconut water maintains the body's potassium and other electrolyte levels.

Diuretics and aquaretics are useful in maintaining kidney health and in treating some forms of kidney disease. The kidneys perform many vital functions and are so important to health that we are born with two of them. They act as a filtering station, garbage dump, processing facility, recycling plant, and regulating agency.

They do this by means of a filtering system that processes about 200 liters of blood a day. The kidneys remove waste products that are continually produced as a result of cellular metabolism. These waste products must be removed from the blood or they quickly accumulate to toxic levels—a condition called uremia or uremic poisoning. During the filtration process, the kidneys selectively remove excess electrolytes, sugar, and hormones, and recycle those that the body still needs. In the process, blood pH is constantly monitored and maintained at a very precise level. The kidneys are also involved in blood pressure regulation. When blood pressure is low, special cells secrete a hormone that initiates constriction of blood vessels and thus raises blood pressure. The kidneys constantly monitor, evaluate, and adjust blood chemistry and, therefore, are essential in maintaining homeostasis.

Any disease or injury that interferes with kidney function is potentially very serious. Kidney failure is one of the most common causes of death. In the US it is the ninth leading cause of death. In Australia it is the seventh. The rates are similar in Europe. Over the past couple of decades, mortality from kidney disease has been increasing by 1.5 percent each year. Part of this may be due to the increasing incidence of other health problems such as heart disease and diabetes, which increase risk of kidney failure.

Kidney failure is the inability of the kidneys to properly process blood and form urine. Diuretics are commonly prescribed to increase urine output in patients whose kidneys fail to produce enough urine, an indicator that harmful waste products are being retained, rather than filtered out by the kidneys.

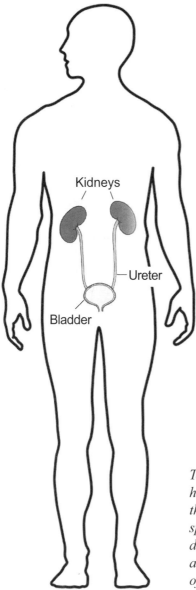

Kidneys

Ureter

Bladder

When kidney function has declined to the point that diuretics are no longer adequate, the use of an artificial kidney machine may be necessary. These machines take over some of the functions of filtering waste from the blood through a process called dialysis. Blood is channeled from an artery in the patient's arm through the dialysis machine, filtered, and pumped back into the patient's arm.

When kidney function is compromised, body chemistry can become unbalanced and a number of health conditions can arise. So keeping the kidneys in good health helps to keep us in good health. Coconut water is like a kidney tonic. It assists the kidneys in producing urine to flush out toxins and excess minerals. It helps to keep these vital organs healthy and

To locate your kidneys, place your hands on your hips with your thumbs almost touching behind the spine. Your kidneys are located underneath your back muscles just above your thumbs on either side of your spine.

functioning properly, thus aiding them in their job of regulating homeostasis. A glass or two of coconut water a day can help to keep your kidneys healthy and your body in balance.

KIDNEY STONES

"I started having kidney stones with my first pregnancy. I would have these spells where I would hurt so badly on one side of my abdomen that I would cry. Tylenol was all I was allowed to take at that time and it didn't even come close to easing the pain. My doctor admitted me to the hospital and found nothing wrong with me and two days later at home I passed two pea-sized stones. What a relief... Stones are the most painful thing I have endured and during a pregnancy it's twice as bad. Anyone that has severe, unexplained pain in the back or abdomen should be checked for renal stones."
—L.J.

"I started having some trouble urinating and kept feeling like I had a urinary tract infection (UTI). I went to the doctor repeatedly only to be told 'No you don't have a UTI.' I finally went to a urologist who ran some tests and said I think you have an over active bladder. Well 2 days later I had to leave work early because my stomach hurt and my lower back hurt. Through the night the pain got worse. My husband, being a nurse and knowing my high pain tolerance gave me a shot of pain medication which helped for awhile. The next morning the pain came back with such intensity that I could not even stand straight. I was crying and thrashing around. My hubby took me to the ER and I begged them to give me something; this pain is worse than giving birth to my kids. At this point I didn't know what was wrong, all I knew was I was in pain and I couldn't urinate. The doctor came in and ordered morphine and finally relief came. I went for a CT scan and the diagnosis was a kidney stone causing a blockage. I went home with lots of pain medicine and a strainer to wait it out. It took me a week to pass the stone."
—Dana

If you have ever passed a kidney stone, you're not likely to forget the experience—it's enough to make a grown man cry. Kidney stones have plagued mankind for generations. They were described by the ancient Egyptians. Today they are a common problem, and in recent years the incidence has been increasing. Many believe that lifestyle, diet, and a lack of fluids are the primary culprits.

High calcium consumption and a diet high in acid forming foods (primarily meat and grains) and low in alkalizing foods (fruits and vegetables) are believed to promote stone formation. Chronic dehydration is also a problem. People who live in hot, dry climates, work in a hot environment, or exercise strenuously without adequately replacing lost fluids experience a higher incidence of kidney stones. According to the US National Institutes of Health, 1 person in 10 develops kidney stones during their lifetime and kidney stone disease accounts for 7-10 of every 1000 hospital admissions. Kidney stones are repeat offenders. Once you have had a kidney stone, there is a 70 percent chance for a reoccurrence.

The kidneys process about 15 gallons (57 liters) of blood every hour. Most of the water and necessary electrolytes are reabsorbed and returned to the bloodstream. Excess water, waste, and minerals are left behind as urine. This is collected into small chambers in the central part of the kidney which drains into the bladder through a tube called the ureter.

If urine production is low or mineral and waste concentration is high, these mineral salts begin to precipitate out of solution and form crystals or "stones" in the central part of the kidney. Most kidney stones are composed of calcium. Calcium is the same mineral that forms limestone, so they are very hard and can be very jagged with sharp edges. When kidney stones take to the road and begin to move, they can scrape and cut the soft lining of the urinary tract, causing intense pain. The larger the stone, the greater the pain. Large stones can even block the flow of urine, causing additional discomfort.

Stones vary in size and shape from tiny particles like grains of sand to large, branched formations filling much of the space in the kidney. The small particles may be voided without a person knowing it. Larger stones may cause intense pain and damage as they travel down the urinary tract.

Frequently, treatment includes drinking larger amounts of water than usual, so that the urine is kept dilute enough to hold all dissolved salts in solution and keep them from crystallizing. Drugs that increase urine output (diuretics) may be used in combination with drugs that dissolve stones to flush the stones out. Lasers and high-energy sound waves have also been used to break up large stones.

A stone that becomes lodged in the urinary tract can become a serious problem and may need to be removed surgically. Obstruction and inflammation in the lower urinary tract may progress to kidney failure.

You are not likely to have any signs or symptoms unless a kidney stone is large, causes a blockage, is associated with an infection, or is being passed. The most common symptom is intense pain that may fluctuate in intensity over periods of five to 15 minutes. The pain usually starts in your back or your side just under or below the edge of your ribs. As the stone moves down the ureter toward your bladder, the pain may radiate to your lower abdomen, groin, and genital area on that side. If the stone stops moving, the pain may stop. Other signs include: bloody, cloudy, or foul-smelling urine; nausea and vomiting; persistent urge to urinate; and if an infection is present, fever and chills.

While small stones may pass without notice, larger ones won't. Stones don't just disappear, they get bigger over time and become more difficult to remove. If you do nothing, they will continue to grow. The reason why most people have a reoccurrence is because they don't do anything to prevent stone formation and new stones develop.

Ways to help prevent stone formation and perhaps even dissolve existing stones is to increase fluid intake in order to increase urine flow and consume more alkalizing foods. Stones like to form in an acidic environment. Alkalizing the urine will help dissolve the stones. Foods containing citric acid, potassium, and magnesium can also help block stone formation. Potassium also improves circulation, dilates blood vessels and improves filtration rate of the kidneys, thus assisting in kidney function.[1] Therefore, a good source of potassium helps the kidneys perform their job. Consuming coconut water can do all of this and it can do it very effectively.

Coconut water has a long tradition for its therapeutic effect on the urinary and reproductive systems. Medical research over the past few

Kidney Stones

Coconut water [in the Philippines] is well known for dissolving kidney stones. My wife used it five years ago for this purpose with success...She drank buko juice (coconut water) of two coconuts a day for about three weeks. The symptoms (pain, blood in urine) disappeared after only two weeks.

G. T.

After having spent many years in the South Pacific Islands of Tonga, we are very much aware of the benefits of coconut. Both my brother and myself have personal experience of the dissolving of kidney stones with very young green coconut water, 2 liters taken over a 24 hour period is all that it takes to dissolve them.

Milton McKenzie

years has shown that coconut water consumption not only prevents kidney stone formation but dissolves them as well.[2] Dr. Eugenio Macalalag, director of the urology department at the Chinese General Hospital in the Philippines, says that coconut water has demonstrated its effectiveness in patients suffering from kidney and urethral stone problems. His patients have even been able to suspend dialysis treatment after regular oral intake of coconut water. In the Philippines, coconut water is commonly known as buko juice. Dr. Macalalag has also reported success in patients by directly infusing the water into the kidneys. He calls the treatment bukolysis. A saying that has now become popular in the Philippines is: "A coconut a day keeps the urologist away."

Coconut water injected through urethral catheters inserted up to where the stones are lodged (bukolysis) has resulted in significant daily decrease in size, disintegration of the stones, and expulsion without the need for surgery. Even by oral intake, coconut water, taken 2 or 3 times a week, has been observed to result in significant size reduction of kidney stones within a short time. Macalalag reports that, of his 1,670 patients who were recurrent stone formers and who took buko therapy, only 13 percent had recurrence of stones in a 10-year period, and the stones were small and passed out easily. Coconut water therapy is so effective that kidney stone patients are spared going though expensive medical procedures. Dr. Macalalag jokingly complains that because of this he suffers from "AIDS" or what he calls "acute income deficiency syndrome."

URINARY TRACT INFECTIONS

"I awoke one day with severe pain. I assumed I had a really bad urinary tract infection. I went to my regular doctor who took a sample of my urine and automatically started me on antibiotics, which gave me a wicked yeast infection. I was now dealing with two painful problems."
—JR

Most urinary tract infections (UTIs) are caused by bacteria. UTIs can involve the urethra, bladder, ureter, or kidneys. We often hear the term cystitis used in reference to UTIs. Cystitis indicates inflammation of the bladder. Inflammation is commonly caused by bacteria, but may also be caused by stones or other factors.

UTIs often appear suddenly. The symptoms can be painful with burning on urination, voiding only a small amount, and maybe the presence of blood in the urine. The bladder or urethra becomes inflamed and irritable. The urine itself may be cloudy because it contains pus or blood and may also have an unpleasant odor. Irritation causes the bladder to send messages to empty with an urgent need to urinate, yet only a trickle may come out. The infection often causes pain in the groin or lower back.

Generally, the infection stays in the bladder, but it can travel up into the kidneys creating a more serious infection. Kidney infections are usually accompanied by chills, high fever, nausea or vomiting, and pain under the rib cage which may radiate to the groin.

The standard treatment for UTIs is antibiotics. One of the problems with taking antibiotics is that they kill bacteria indiscriminately so that even the good bacteria in the digestive tract fall prey to them. Intestinal bacteria are important because they synthesize many important vitamins.

They also prevent the overgrowth of harmful organisms such as candida. Candida is a yeast—a single celled fungus—so it is not harmed by antibiotics. When we take antibiotics and kill off the friendly bacteria, Candida is allowed to grow without restraint, often resulting in a systemic and/or localized candida infection. So you can end up trading a bacterial infection for a yeast infection.

A healthy bladder normally has a sterile environment. The body's natural defenses keep it that way. The antimicrobial surface of the bladder, the removal of bacteria during urination, and urine pH are normally unsuitable for the growth of troublesome bacteria. Bacteria are normally washed away during urination. Generous fluid intake, around 8 glasses of water a day, ensures efficient flushing. Drinking plenty of fluids also dilutes the urine, lowering the concentration of bacteria that might be present.

UTIs are not normally life threatening and the body's immune system can fend off the attack. Often, simply increasing fluid intake and urination is enough to dilute and flush the infection away. An effective way to do this is with aquaretic herbs and foods such as coconut water.

We do not live in a sterile world. Bacteria that can infect the urinary tract are around us all the time. Some people are more prone to infections than others. Part of the reason is diet and lifestyle. When bacteria find a suitable environment, they quickly reproduce and an infection results. Our bodies are capable of defending themselves but we need to supply them with good nutrition and plenty of fluids for this to happen.

Drinking the juice from one or two green coconuts daily can be helpful in fighting off an active UTI. One average-size coconut contains from 12-16 ounces of water. With adequate plain water consumption, about 12 ounces of coconut water a day is generally enough to prevent further infections.

EDEMA

If you were watching an old Western on television, you might see the town doctor lament that one of his patients is suffering from dropsy. Dropsy is an older term for what we know today as edema. Edema is swelling caused by the accumulation of excess fluid. Although not an

94

illness in itself, it is a sign or symptom of a more serious problem such as heart failure or kidney disease.

Our cells are bathed in a sea of fluid. This fluid seeps out from the bloodstream through the capillaries, bringing with it oxygen and nutrients to feed the cells. Oxygen is exchanged for carbon dioxide and the fluid reenters the bloodstream through the capillaries. In this way all the cells of the body are nourished and metabolic waste removed. The kidneys regulate the amount of water that flows through the bloodstream and around our cells.

Edema occurs when excess fluid accumulates in the spaces between the cells. Edema of the ankles and feet is quite common. People who are on their feet a lot may have puffy ankles. This is not a serious condition and may be corrected simply by resting with the feet elevated. Severe or chronic swelling may be a sign that something is seriously wrong. The kidneys are unable to properly regulate body fluids or electrolyte levels.

The standard treatment for edema involves eating a low sodium diet (sodium increases water retention) and taking diuretics. For mild cases, coconut water can be of help by removing excess fluid. Rest and elevation are useful too. Sometimes edema is so mild it is difficult to see. A simple way of identifying edema when it isn't obvious is to press your finger into the skin; if it is swollen it will make an indentation that slowly flattens out as the fluid seeps back.

CARDIOVASCULAR DISEASE
Coconut Water and Heart Disease

Cardiovascular disease is scary. To most of us it means heart disease, and heart disease kills. It is the number one cause of death worldwide. We all have family members or acquaintances who have died as a result of heart disease. Cardiovascular disease actually involves any problem that affects the heart or circulatory system. The clogging of the arteries with plaque, high blood pressure, heart attacks, and strokes are conditions associated with cardiovascular disease.

High blood pressure is of concern to doctors because it causes stress within the arteries which may lead to minute injuries and chronic inflammation—conditions that promote the processes that lead to the development of plaque or atherosclerosis. Cholesterol, scar tissue, calcium, and blood clots accumulate at the damaged site in the artery to form plaque. Plaque in arteries blocks blood flow to vital organs such as the heart and brain.

High blood pressure is not only harmful to the arteries but is also hard on the kidneys. The delicate filtering tissues of the kidney can be permanently damaged by excessive blood pressure. When this happens, the kidney's ability to filter waste and produce urine is compromised. The kidneys help to regulate blood pressure yet, ironically, high blood pressure can dampen the kidney's ability to perform this function. Diuretics or preferably aquaretics can be useful in reducing blood pressure and thus lower risk of heart and kidney disease.

Coconut water in many respects can be viewed as a heart tonic. When researchers were experimenting with the use of coconut water as an intravenous fluid, they paid particular attention to how the water affected cardiovascular health. If coconut water was harmful to the heart or arteries, it would become very evident when the water was pumped directly into the bloodstream.

In the early days of intravenous therapy, doctors discovered that when patients were given potassium-rich IV saline solutions to treat potassium deficiency, the process required intense monitoring. The addition of the potassium predisposed patients to ventricular tachycardia—a potentially lethal disruption of the normal heart beat. Since coconut water was high in potassium, researchers looked very closely at how it affected the heart. Apparently, the electrolyte balance of coconut water is such that there is no detrimental effect on the heart or the circulatory system as a whole. Dr. Benjamin Eiseman in his pioneering work on IV coconut water therapy states, "Cardiac irregularities, palpitation, and hypotension did not attend any infusions, although we carefully looked for them."[3] His study involved 157 individuals who received coconut water intravenously. Eiseman could find no evidence that the arteries were harmed in any way. In an earlier study he stated, "After infusion, regardless of the rate or size of vein employed, we found no evidence of thrombophlebitis or thrombosis."[4] So there was no inflammation or abnormal clotting and no irregularities in heart function. This has since been confirmed by other researchers.

Atherosclerosis and Cholesterol

What all this proves is that coconut water is not harmful to the cardiovascular system. But that is not the end of the story. Coconut water apparently isn't just an innocent bystander either; it can take an active role in protecting the heart and arteries from disease. A study by Chinese researchers demonstrated that coconut water inhibited the formation of atherosclerosis (arterial plaque), thus keeping the arteries healthy and open.[5]

Although quails were used in this study, it provides valuable information on how coconut water can protect us from atherosclerosis and heart disease. The researchers fed the animals a special fatty diet to quickly induce atherosclerosis. The diet in some of the animals was supplemented with 20 ml of coconut water to see what effect, if any, it would have on blood lipid levels. The results were intriguing. HDL cholesterol levels increased by an amazing 46.2 percent. HDL cholesterol is known as the "good" cholesterol because it lowers the risk of heart disease and atherosclerosis. The higher the HDL the better, so a 46.2 percent increase signifies a substantial reduction in heart disease risk. Liver total cholesterol levels were reduced by 26.3 percent and the index of atherosclerosis was reduced by 41.1 percent.

A similar study was conducted by researchers in India. In this study rats were used. The animals were fed a high cholesterol atherogenic diet to increase cholesterol levels and promote atherosclerosis. The animals were given both young and mature coconut water at a dose level of 4 ml/100g of body weight. The cholesterol feeding caused a marked increase in total cholesterol and LDL (bad) cholesterol. The researchers noted coconut water "counteracts" the increase in total and LDL cholesterol, reduced the amount of cholesterol deposited in the liver and aorta of the animals, and increased dilation of the arteries, allowing blood to flow more freely.[6] This study demonstrated that both young and mature coconut water are beneficial in preventing atherosclerosis and reducing risk of heart disease.

High Blood Pressure

High blood pressure is one of the primary risk factors associated with heart disease. Its association is strong because it can be actively involved in the development of atherosclerosis. As noted earlier in this chapter, increasing the production of urine can help reduce blood pressure. Coconut water can do this. The minerals potassium and magnesium are also known to help reduce blood pressure, as you have seen in Chapter 4. Coconut water is high in both of these. Therefore, it is no wonder that coconut water can be useful in lowering high blood pressure. Studies confirm this. For example, in one study 28 volunteers with high blood pressure consumed coconut water for a two week period. In that short amount of time blood pressure declined in 71 percent of the participants.[7] This study showed how coconut water can lower high blood pressure. Drinking coconut water on a regular basis may be a good way to lower elevated blood pressure and keep it under control.

The use of diuretics is recognized as an effective means to reduce high blood pressure, and consequently, reduce risk of heart disease. The Joint National Committee and the World Health Organization recommend diuretics as the first-line therapy for uncomplicated hypertension. This recommendation is based on multiple clinical studies demonstrating the effectiveness of diuretics in reducing high blood pressure and reducing stress on the heart.[8-9]

Ever since the Veterans Administration study in the 1970s, studies have documented that diuretic-based therapy reduces the risk of stroke and heart attacks and cardiovascular morbidity and mortality.[10-11]

A major study known as the Systolic Hypertension in the Elderly Program (SHEP) used a diuretic to treat high blood pressure. At the end of five years the study showed that lowering blood pressure yielded a statistically significant reduction in adverse events related to coronary heart disease, congestive heart failure, and overall cardiovascular disease.[12]

Another similar study was the Syst-Eur trial.[12] This study involved 4,650 subjects. It showed that strokes, heart failure, and heart attacks declined by a total of 31 percent in those taking diuretics. The study was stopped after just two years because it was deemed unethical to continue giving one group placebos when the data showed a clear advantage in the treatment group.

Coconut water's aquaretic effect is only one way in which it can lower high blood pressure. Another way is the effect it has on blood vessel dilation. The amino acids in coconut water, especially arginine, participate in chemical reactions that stimulate blood vessel dilation, thus opening them up and allowing a greater volume of blood to flow.[14-15] Wider blood vessels means lower blood pressure and reduced risk of heart attack.

Heart Failure

One common form of heart disease is heart failure, a condition in which the heart is weakened to the point that it is unable to pump the blood rapidly enough to maintain the normal rate of circulation. Although the term "heart failure" sounds like a fatal irreversible condition, it is usually treatable and patients can survive for years afterwards. Many people are living with some degree of heart failure without even knowing it.

Causes of heart failure include chronic high blood pressure, coronary heart disease, a previous heart attack that has weakened the heart, and less commonly, congenital birth defects of the heart valves.

Whatever the cause, the heart fails to empty completely with each contraction or has difficulty accepting blood returning from the lungs. The retained blood creates a back pressure that causes the lungs to become congested with blood. This, in turn, leads to pulmonary edema (excess fluid in the lungs), of which the main symptom is shortness of breath. The heart may also become congested, pushing the blood backwards into the veins. Fluid may escape from the veins into the tissues, causing congestion in the intestines, indigestion, heartburn, and swelling in the ankles and feet.

The basic treatment for heart failure is a low salt diet and diuretics to rid the body of excess fluid and reduce blood volume, which eases the workload on the heart. Vasodilator drugs may also be prescribed, which open the blood vessels to allow easier flow of blood. These measures usually bring about a significant improvement within a few days.

Coconut water can be an excellent aid in preventing heart failure. Its aquaretic effect removes excess fluid and its potassium and magnesium help dilate blood vessels to allow easier blood flow.

An interesting study with coconut water was published by researchers in India in 1956.[16] While studying the electrolyte composition of coconut water their interest was aroused by its possible use in treating congestive heart failure. Although they were aware that coconut water was traditionally used as a diuretic, to their knowledge it had not been studied when used in large quantities or as the sole item in the diet.

In this study 10 hospitalized heart failure patients were divided into two equal groups. The first group received on average 60 fluid ounces of young coconut water, plus two cups (16 ounces total) of tea daily. They received no other food or fluids. The second group was given the standard treatment for heart failure at that time. Both groups received an equal amount of fluids.

The patients were put on the program for five days. Urinary output for those receiving the coconut water peaked on about the third day and then tapered off. Weight loss due to removal of excess water ranged from 16-29 pounds over the five day period. All of the patients in this group felt better within five days. In three of the cases the improvement was so rapid that the researchers noted that "therapy on the fifth day was superfluous." Although the patients received large quantities of coconut water almost exclusively, no toxic or adverse effects were observed. These patients, however, showed a desire to eat food before the fifth day, reflecting their rapid clinical improvement.

In the group that received the standard treatment, urinary output was sporadic and of lesser volume. Except for two cases, there was no significant weight loss (i.e., water loss). None of the patients in the coconut water group required supplementary therapy but three patients in this group required mercurial injections to stimulate diuresis.

By comparison, the coconut water group demonstrated much faster improvement without the need of potentially toxic drugs.

In summary, coconut water has no known harmful effects on the cardiovascular system. It appears to improve cholesterol levels, prevent atherosclerosis, keep blood vessels open, normalize blood pressure, and remove excess fluids that stress the heart and other organs. In short, coconut water acts as a health tonic, good for the heart.

EYE HEALTH

To have a doctor say that you are losing your vision is a scary experience. Eyesight is one of our most cherished senses. Maintaining good vision is a high priority. Many visual problems can be avoided with a little preventative care. Glaucoma and cataracts are two such conditions.

Glaucoma is a dreaded disease because it can lead to total and permanent blindness. Glaucoma occurs when fluid pressure within the eyeball becomes abnormally high, causing damage to tiny blood vessels and the optic nerve. Between 2-3 million people in the United States have glaucoma, and 120,000 of these are legally blind as a result. It is the leading cause of preventable blindness in the United States. The risk of glaucoma increases dramatically with age.

Glaucoma is sneaky. About half of the people who are affected are unaware of it. There are no symptoms in the early stage, and progression is so slow that small changes in vision go undetected. The first symptom is often unnoticeable blind spots at the edges of the field of vision. As the disease progresses, peripheral vision is gradually lost, progressing to tunnel vision, and then to blindness. Sight lost from glaucoma cannot be restored. The only way to detect early stage glaucoma is with an eye exam.

Glaucoma is basically a plumbing problem. Water is constantly entering and leaving the eyeball. This fluid brings in nutrients and carries away waste. Normally the rate that fluid comes into the eye equals the amount leaving. However, if water enters the eyeball quicker than it can exit, fluid pressure begins to build. As the pressure increases, the force against the inside of the eyeball increases. This pressure cuts off the blood circulation to tiny blood vessels and capillaries that feed the optic nerve. Deprived of adequate blood circulation, the optic nerve gradually dies.

There is no cure for glaucoma; all that can be done is to prevent it from worsening. Treatment consists of putting medication in the eye to reduce fluid flow into the eye or increase fluid removal. Medicated eye drops must be used on a regular basis to keep the fluid pressure under control. If treatment is continued throughout life, vision will be preserved in most cases.

Although the exact cause of fluid buildup in the eye is unknown, water retention is involved. Therefore, diuretics have been useful in reducing eye fluid pressure. With that in mind, coconut water may be useful in managing or preventing this condition. The few studies that have been done in this regard have shown that coconut water is effective

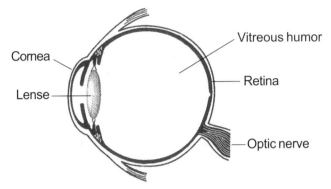

The eye is filled with a watery gel called vitreous humor. Too much of this fluid causes excessive pressures which can lead to glaucoma.

in reducing fluid pressure in the eyes. Fluid pressure is significantly reduced by drinking coconut water, with the effect lasting for at least 2½ hours, which currently is the maximum period of time investigated by researchers.[17]

Cataract is another common vision problem. Cataract is basically the clouding of the lens of the eye. It is usually associated with aging. Most people develop some clouding of the lens after the age of 60. About 50 percent of people aged 65-74, and about 70 percent of those 75 and older, have cataracts that affect their vision. Cataract can occur in either or both eyes. It does not spread from one eye to the other.

In a normal eye, light passes through the transparent lens and is focused on the retina. The retina is the light-sensitive tissue at the back of the eye. Once it reaches the retina, light is changed into nerve signals that are sent to the brain. The lens must be clear for the retina to receive a sharp image. If the lens is cloudy from a cataract, the image is blurred.

The lens is made of mostly water and protein. The protein is arranged in a precise way that keeps the lens clear and allows light to pass through. As we age, some of the protein may clump together and start to cloud small areas of the lens, producing cataracts. Over time, the cataract may grow larger and cloud more of the lens, making it harder to see.

The most common symptoms of cataract are: cloudy or blurry vision, loss of color intensity, glare (headlights or sunlight may appear too bright), halos around lights, poor night vision, double vision, and frequent changes in eyeglass prescription. If cataracts become so severe that they interfere with daily activities such as driving or reading, they are corrected through surgery. Surgery involves removing the affected lens and replacing it with an artificial lens.

Another possible treatment for cataracts involves the use of coconut water. Some years ago one of my patients told me about a treatment for cataracts she found in a book by noted herbalist John Heinerman. In the book he advised the patient to lie down and put several drops of fresh coconut water into the eyes, then apply a hot damp washcloth over the eyes for about 10 minutes.

According to Heinerman even one application is enough to get significant improvement. My patient had cataracts, so she tried it on herself and reported that it worked! I have mentioned this to others since then and they too have reported positive results. It doesn't always work with only one application, it may require several to gain improvement.

More recently I ran across an interesting incident which dramatically illustrates the potential benefit coconut water may have in treating cataract. I'll let Marjie tell the story in her own words.

"We discovered this by accident while on a cruise ship (years ago). A few of us were on an island day trip and wanted to get off the beaten tourist's path so we hired a bus and driver to take us to the opposite side of the island (only 10 of us on that big bus). A man and his wife were taking the cruise as a sort of last hoorah before her scheduled cataract surgery, we later found out. Anyway, there was a beautiful beach with coconuts laying everywhere and we got thirsty, but there was no drinking water. So we decided to open up some coconuts to quench our dry throats. We found a local with a big machete and through sign language we convinced him to open coconuts for us. The woman with the cataracts got splashed in one eye by the coconut juice, and it burned a bit. We were all digging through everything we had for something to relieve her eye 'injury.' All we came up with was one moist washcloth. Her husband wiped her eye and placed the washcloth over it. About 10 minutes later she announced we should head back to the ship. We did. The next morning at breakfast she said that her eye was much better and that she could see very well. We examined her eye closely and could not see any signs of the cataract, which was quite obvious the day before. She said she wished she had gotten splashed in both eyes. Then the idea dawned on us to 'splash' her other eye. We did that very day as soon as we got ashore and also repeated the other eye too. This time we were prepared. We went to the local market, grabbed a coconut, opened it, and strained it through a washcloth into a plastic cup, dribbled the juice into both eyes, placed a warm washcloth over both eyes, waited 10 minutes, and the rest is history. She went to her MD upon returning stateside—no cataracts and no surgery."

What is it in coconut water that may have an effect on cataracts? Coconut water contains antioxidants as well as magnesium, potassium and other minerals and enzymes which may un-denature or relax the lens proteins, allowing them to realign and become transparent again. I suspect that for this procedure to work as well as reported, *fresh* coconut water is needed.

Coconut water may be an ideal eyewash or eye drop solution. If it can heal the damage caused by cataract, it may have other beneficial effects on eye health as well. Using it regularly may be an excellent way to prevent cataract, glaucoma, and perhaps other eye problems.

CONSTIPATION

Sometimes simply drinking coconut water will bring noticeable beneficial changes. I advised a friend that he should drink more fluids during the day and casually mentioned coconut water as a good hydration beverage. He showed interest so I gave him some bottled coconut water to take home. I met him again a few days later. "Where did you get that coconut water?" he asked eagerly. "I want more." Surprised by his enthusiastic reaction, I asked what had inspired his interest. He explained that drinking about 11 ounces a day (the amount in each of the containers I gave him) softened his stools, relieving his chronic constipation and easing the pain he experiences from hemorrhoids. He promptly went out and purchased six cases of coconut water. He didn't want to risk not having any on hand if later the store happened to be sold out. He now drinks at least 11 ounces of coconut water daily. I had not mentioned to him that the water was useful for this purpose or any health condition. I only indicated that it was good for hydration.

The laxative effect of coconut water is well known in the tropics. When I say it has a "laxative" effect, I don't mean it will cause diarrhea; it simply softens the stools and increases the urge for relief. How much is needed to loosen the stool? This is an individual issue. I can drink the water from at least eight coconuts in a single day and not have an issue with overusing the bathroom. Its effect may be more noticeable in some people than it is in others.

Your state of hydration also affects the way your body responds. Chronic dehydration and constipation go hand-in-hand. If you want to use coconut water as an aid for constipation, you also need to keep well hydrated by drinking plenty of plain water during the day. Remember the 6-8 glasses of water a day rule and include a glass or two of coconut water. More coconut water can be added if necessary.

DIABETES

One of the characteristics of diabetes is poor blood circulation and a tendency to develop atherosclerosis. About 73 percent of adults with diabetes also have high blood pressure. Both diabetes and high blood pressure are major risk factors for heart disease. When both are present, the risk significantly increases. Heart disease is the primary cause of death in diabetics. Lowering blood pressure and reducing the processes that promote atherosclerosis can significantly improve the health of someone with diabetes.

In recent years, diuretics have gained much attention in the research community in protecting diabetics from the consequences of heart and kidney diseases. A series of studies have been published as a result of the Antihypertensive and Lipid-Lowering Treatment to Prevent Heart Attack Trial (ALLHAT). One aspect of this study was to evaluate the effectiveness of the three major classes of medication—diuretics, ACE-inhibitors, and calcium channel blockers—used in reducing high blood pressure and protecting against heart attack and kidney disease.[18] The study involved a total 42,418 participants, all with high blood pressure, including many diabetics and those with mildly elevated fasting glucose (pre-diabetics). Other studies have demonstrated the usefulness of diuretics in treating high blood pressure in non-diabetics. This study included diabetics. It was found that diuretics were more protective than the other drugs against congestive heart failure, lowering high blood pressure, preventing heart attacks and strokes, and more protective against death due to *all* causes. These results were seen in both diabetic and non-diabetic subjects.

One of the conclusions reached by the researchers is that diuretics offer an effective, inexpensive, and simple means of reducing the risks associated with diabetes. Aquaretics such as coconut water offer a simple means by which diabetics and pre-diabetics can help ward off complications associated with this disease.

Besides the diuretic effect, coconut water has another possible benefit for diabetics. Although it tastes sweet, it does not have the detrimental effect on blood sugar levels that other fruit juices have. Coconut water is probably similar in composition to coconut sap which feeds the growing coconuts. Coconut sap is often dehydrated to remove the moisture and concentrate the sugar. Coconut sugar has a glycemic index of only 35. The glycemic index is an indicator that measures how foods affect blood sugar. An index of 70 and more is high, 55-70 is medium, and below 55 is low. So 35 is very low. In comparison, Gatorade has an index of 78, white bread 70, and a banana 56. The sweetness in coconut water comes from a combination of fructose, glucose, sucrose, inulin, and sorbitol. The glycemic index of fructose is only 22 and that of inulin and sorbitol is zero. So it is not surprising that coconut water does not spike blood sugar like other fruit juices.

Inulin, one of the carbohydrates that adds sweetness to coconut water, is interesting. Although the name is similar to insulin, the two are completely different and have no connection with one another. Insulin is a hormone, while inulin is a fructooligosaccharide—a string of fructose molecules liked together with a glucose molecule at the end. Nutritionally it is considered a dietary fiber because we don't have enzymes that can break it up into smaller units. Dietary fiber helps to regulate blood sugar, improves digestion, and nutriment absorption. Friendly gut bacteria feed on it, which help to keep our internal environment healthy. A liter of coconut water contains about 150 mg of inulin.

There is a little over 1 gram of total carbohydrate/sugar per ounce of coconut water. Despite the sugar content, some diabetics report improvement in blood sugar levels when they start drinking coconut water. Audrey L. was always having trouble keeping her blood sugar under control even though she carefully watched what she ate. After every meal, her blood sugar would rise and she would routinely take insulin to keep it under control. She had begun to use coconut oil in her diet and thought she might also try adding coconut water. The results surprised her.

"I am sharing my experience with this wonderful discovery," says Audrey. "Now, please, don't think I am playing doctor, but I have to say something about my own personal experience with coconut juice…I am a diabetic. I am very insulin dependent. Since drinking the coconut water, and it is high carb for me, 29 carbs per drink, my blood glucose is staying down! I drink a can of it along with my meal, and do my insulin and an hour later, test, and my blood glucose is in the normal range. I haven't changed the dosage of my insulin at all either!…This is the third week of the water and oil and so far so good."

One of the reasons why coconut water is of benefit in controlling blood sugar is because it contains arginine, an amino acid that helps moderate sugar absorption.[19] Arginine also improves insulin sensitivity so that blood sugar is more readily transported from the bloodstream into the cells.[20]

Another benefit with arginine is that it opens up the arteries, an important issue to diabetics. One of the major characteristics of diabetes is poor circulation. Complications commonly associated with diabetes such as heart attacks, blindness, kidney failure, leg ulcers (peripheral vascular disease), and slow wound healing are all a consequence of poor blood circulation. Arginine improves blood circulation thus protecting against these conditions.

The benefits of arginine are so remarkable that the following section takes a closer look at how it affects health.

ARGININE

Some of the observed, traditional, and clinical benefits associated with coconut water are probably associated with the amino acid content of the water. Amino acids are the molecular building blocks for proteins. They are involved in tissue repair and building and for the synthesis of hormones and enzymes. There are 20 amino acids in our foods that are important to human health. Of this number nine are considered essential because they cannot be synthesized from any of the others. Coconut water contains 18 of the 20 amino acids, including all nine of the essential ones. One amino acid in particular—arginine—is present in relatively high amounts, an important issue because of the way it can influence health. The amount of arginine isn't huge in comparison to high protein foods such as eggs or beef, but is apparently significant enough to have many positive effects.

Arginine is considered a conditionally essential amino acid. While it is absolutely essential for good health, it can be synthesized, if necessary, from other essential amino acids. However, under some conditions, this process may be too slow to fully meet needs, and a deficiency can exist. Therefore, it is considered semi-essential. Conditions that can lead to arginine deficiency are an unbalanced diet, protein deficiency, malnutrition, rapid growth, intense physical stress, injury, or infection.

Arginine performs many vital functions in the body. It is essential for the breakdown of protein and the production of urea in urine. It plays a role in protein synthesis and is crucial during periods of rapid growth, in the healing of wounds and injuries, and in the prevention of wasting in people with critical illness. It affects the production and secretion of human growth hormones, strengthens the immune system, enhances fertility, inhibits the growth of certain cancers, improves liver function, and supports heart and circulatory health. In athletes it is reported to enhance muscle mass and reduce body fat. Its benefits are so numerous that it is often sold as a dietary supplement.

Our bodies use arginine in the production of nitric oxide (NO), which regulates blood vessel dilation. When blood vessels dilate, blood flow increases and stress on the heart decreases. For this reason, researchers believe arginine may be useful in the treatment of a number of conditions involving poor circulation such as angina, atherosclerosis, heart failure, peripheral vascular disease, erectile dysfunction, and vascular headache. Arginine given orally or intravenously has been shown to dilate blood vessels, inhibit platelet sticking, lower blood pressure, increase blood flow, and prevent and even reverse atherosclerosis.[21]

Most of the studies demonstrating the benefits of arginine use large amounts—4, 5, 10 grams, or more a day. The amount you would get from drinking the water from a fresh coconut would generally be about a half gram. The question one might ask is whether the amount of arginine in coconut water is enough to bring about noticeable changes in health? The answer apparently is "yes." Perhaps the presence of other amino acids or nutrients enhance the effects of arginine. Many of the benefits associated with coconut water are similar to those credited to arginine.

Studies have shown that the topical application of arginine can enhance wound healing and improve skin conditions such as dermatitis and dry skin.[22-23] It has also been reported to be useful in healing ulcers, combating hair loss, and improving libido. The reasoning behind the topical use of arginine is that it relaxes blood vessels near the surface of the skin, enhancing blood flow to tissues. Perhaps this is one reason why coconut water has been used traditionally as a topical ointment for ulcers, boils, and skin infections. It may also explain why it has been reported to help with cataracts.

Arginine Content in Beverages

	(g/100 gram portion)
Coconut Water	.118
Orange Juice	.047
Apple Juice	.006
Carrot Juice	.093
Whole Milk	.075
Grape Juice	.047
Tomato Juice	.015
Watermelon	.059
Coffee, black	0
Gatorade	0
ORS	0

One cup of coconut water contains .283 grams of arginine.

Vomiting

Since September I have been drinking one coconut a day and sometimes two. I have found that my energy level has increased and my hair looks better. Recently, I had a severe migraine and was vomiting. I could not hold anything down for the whole day, not even water. By the end of the day I was very thirsty and weak. Then I remembered that since coconut water has electrolytes, vitamins, and trace minerals, I should give it a try. To my surprise, I immediately felt better and my vomiting stopped. Since then, I have had a similar experience and again it had helped me. So this is no coincidence.

Wendy Y.

Yeast Infection

I have been buying coconuts this past week and eating almost half a coconut a day now. I love the coconut water! I had a yeast infection for almost two weeks, and it is almost gone. I started eating the coconut and water about four days ago, and that's when I started to notice that the infection was dissipating.

S.P.

Arginine exerts a positive effect on the immune system, primarily by stimulating thymus activity and supporting lymphocyte (white blood cell) production. Arginine inhibits the growth of tumors by enhancing the efficiency of the immune system. Arginine aids in liver detoxification by neutralizing ammonia, a waste byproduct of protein metabolism. Arginine stimulates the release of human growth hormones which help in muscle building, leading to increased muscle strength and tone, enhances fat metabolism, and is reported to have anti-aging and recuperative effects. It is also being investigated as a means to treat sterility and libido, particularly in men, but even women report positive effects.

Young coconut water has long been noted as an aphrodisiac. It enhances both male and female libido and fertility. This effect is undoubtedly due, at least in part, to the arginine in the water. The ability of coconut water to rehydrate the body faster than plain water or commercial rehydration fluids may be due, in part, to the dilating effect of arginine on the blood vessels. The rapid improvement in cholera victims may be due to both the rehydrating effect and the enhancement of the immune system. The wound healing ability of arginine and the release of growth hormones may have contributed to the rapid recovery of the stroke patient in the Atoifi Hospital, described in Chapter 2. Whether arginine is responsible for all of these effects or not, the fact is that the combination of nutrients in coconut water work synergistically together to improve health in numerous ways.

LIVING ENERGY

What does a marathon runner, a race car, a bicycle, and a computer all have in common? They all require energy to function. Energy is the driving force behind all movement or change. Energy is defined as the ability to cause matter to move or change. There are many forms of energy such as gravitational, magnetic, electrical, nuclear, thermal (heat), radiant (sunlight), elastic, etc. A fundamental law of physics, known as the Law of Conservation of Energy, states that energy cannot be created or destroyed, although it can change from one form to another. An electric stove, for instance, converts electrical energy into thermal energy to cook foods. Plants convert radiant energy from the sun into chemical energy for growth.

The energy from the food that you eat is stored in your body as chemical energy until you use it. It is then converted into heat and motion. Our bodies are subjected to and utilize all forms of energy. These forms of energy can have a powerful influence on us physically, chemically, and psychologically, which affects our health. For this reason, an entire branch of medicine has developed called *energy medicine* that utilizes various forms of energy to treat sickness. A simple example would be using energy in the form of heat to relax muscles and increase blood flow. Another example is the use of electricity to accelerate the body's ability to nit broken bones back together. Energy from heat, electricity, frequencies, light, magnets, and so forth are used in energy medicine to cause changes in the body that facilitate healing.

Another form of energy that is harder to define, but is nonetheless real, is the energy that identifies all life. It is the innate energy inside all living matter. It is what separates inanimate objects from living organisms. This energy is known by different names. We often refer to it as the life force or vital energy. It is called *chi* in China, *qi* in Japan, and *doshas* in India. Humans, animals, plants, and even cells cannot function without this living energy. Without this energy there would be no life.

Eating fresh, raw (living) foods is no doubt healthier than eating highly processed foods. We would all do better if we ate more fresh fruit and vegetables and less chicken nuggets and French fries. Some people feel that "living" foods are healthier, not only because the nutrients are fresh, but because they also include the living energies of the foods themselves. This energy is believed to complement or boost our own vital energy and thus improve health. We know from energy medicine that other forms of energy can have a dramatic affect on health. So, perhaps living energies can too. Whether this is true or not, I don't know, but it is an interesting concept. Let's take a look at how this idea relates to coconuts.

Cells are living organisms just as much as you or I are. They have a covering or skin called a cell membrane (if it's an animal cell) or cell wall (if it's a plant cell) filled with liquid and organelles. Organelles are the cell's organs. The nucleus, which contains the cell's DNA is like the brain. It controls the cell's actions and lifecycle. The fluid or cytoplasm is like the cell's blood. The cytoplasm and organelles together are referred to as the protoplasm.

As living organisms, they have "living" energy. Remember, energy involves movement. Living cells can grow and reproduce, and in some cases are capable of independent movement. The fluid inside cells is dynamic, it moves. In many plants this movement is very pronounced and is called cytoplasmic streaming. As long as the cell is alive the fluid constantly flows in a circular motion, somewhat analogous to blood moving in our bodies.

When you look at most plant cells, the largest organelle is the vacuole. The vacuole is a cavity filled with nonliving plant sap. The sap is composed mostly of water containing sugars, salts, organic acids, pigments, etc. The vacuole may take up almost the entire space inside the cell, leaving only a small portion for the protoplasm. Much of the color of fruits and vegetables come from pigments inside the vacuole. For instance, the blues and reds of radishes, grapes, plums, and cherries and the colors in flowers come from these pigments.

When you make juice from an apple or orange you need to crush all the cells in the fruit to extract the liquid. The resulting fluid no longer functions as a living organism. It's like squeezing the juice out of a fish; the fish juice isn't alive. Neither is the fruit juice. Also, the vast majority of fruit and vegetable juices comes from the contents of the vacuole—the nonliving portion of the cell. Although the resulting juice may be fresh and loaded with nutritious vitamins and minerals, it is not living. It no longer possesses living energy.

The juice from the coconut is different. It is more than just a broth of nutrients. It is living tissue. Coconut water is cell protoplasm—the living material inside cells.

Coconut water is filled with cell organelles, including nuclei. What is interesting about the cells which make up coconut water is that they do not have individual cell walls like most other plant cells. The nuclei and organelles are all a part of the same protoplasm. The coconut shell, in essence, serves as one big cell wall. As the coconut matures, the nuclei migrate to and attach themselves to the shell wall. Here cell walls start to form around each of the nuclei and the coconut water transforms into coconut meat. This is the white meat you see along the inside of the shell when you open a mature coconut.

Coconut water is intracellular fluid. It is interesting that the chemical content of coconut water in many ways is similar to human intracellular fluid. Coconut water contains the same electrolytes as human cells. Like human cells it also contains sugars, amino acids, enzymes, and hormones. There is one more very important similarity. *Both are living tissues*.

Coconut water is composed of a colony of living cells. Like other living tissue, the water is programmed for self-preservation, propagation, and restoration or healing. It is more than just a juice. It is a healing liquid with living energy.

There is power is living tissue—the power to heal and to propagate. Horticulturists learned centuries ago that they could cut off a living branch of one plant and graft it into the stem of another plant and it would continue to grow and produce fruit. Human and animal tissues can also be grafted. Organ transplants and blood infusions are commonplace. Lives are saved.

Just like a blood transfusion from one living organism to another, when you drink the juice from a fresh coconut it is almost like getting a blood transfusion. The living fluid from the coconut is transferred directly to you.

The fact that coconut water can be used successfully as an intravenous fluid may, in part, be because it is living tissue, unlike commercial saline solutions. This may be the reason for many of the health benefits attributed to it that cannot be fully explained by its chemical and nutritional properties alone. From what we have seen, it appears that coconut water enhances the healing energies of our own body. Whether it is the life energy, the nutritional profile, the hormones, or some other factor yet to be identified, the fact is coconut water promotes good health.

6

The Youth Solution

IN SEARCH OF THE FOUNTAIN OF YOUTH

Stories of the fountain of youth have been told since the time of Alexander the Great (356-323 BC). Legend has it that drinking the water from the fountain restores youth, cures disease, and prolongs life. Throughout the years, many adventurers have searched in vain for this mysterious spring. In Europe interest in the fountain peaked during the Renaissance as adventurers roamed the globe exploring new lands.

Spanish explorer Juan Ponce De Leon (1460-1521) is the most famous in this respect. Ponce De Leon was with Christopher Columbus in his early explorations of the Americas. Rumor had it that the fountain was located on an island in the Caribbean. He searched for many years in the Caribbean and ventured up into Florida, thinking it to be an island. Here he came into conflict with the natives and was fatally wounded in battle. He died never having found the fabled fountain.

Ironically, the fountain of youth Ponce De Leon sought for so many years was staring him in the face the entire time. The famed water, as suspected, could be found on an island, but was not from a spring coming out of the ground. It was up in the air, inside the shells of the coconuts growing abundantly everywhere around him. While a supernatural water having the power to transform an old person into a younger one is pure fiction, coconut water is probably the closest thing to it. It can nourish the body and in many cases restore health, which in itself can be considered a youth-enhancing effect. But research shows it can also slow the aging process and, in some cases, even reverse some of the effects of aging. In this respect, coconut water is a fountain of youth.

THE MIRACLE OF PHYTOCHEMICALS

"Phyto" means plant and "phytochemicals" refers to the natural chemicals in plants. There are thousands of phytochemicals in the plant kingdom. Some are classified as nutrients such as vitamins and carotenoids; some function as plant pigments like chlorophyll (green), lycopene (red), and beta-carotene (yellow); others like phytohormones, are involved in plant growth and development. All of these can have an effect on us.

Both plants and animals have hormones. Hormones are chemical messengers that regulate growth, function, and metabolism. In the human body thyroid hormones regulate body temperature and metabolism. Human growth hormones regulate our growth and development. Pancreatic hormones balance blood sugar levels. Sex hormones control sexual development, differentiation, and function. Hormones govern just about every aspect of our lives.

Plant hormones regulate cell division, root growth, shoot production, and flowering. Many plant hormones are chemically very similar to animal and human hormones. Consequently, plant hormones can have a similar affect on the function of our bodies as do our own hormones.

Phytoestrogens, for example, are chemicals in plants that mimic the human sex hormone estrogen. Isoflavones in soybeans and lignans in flaxseed are two common phytoesterogens.

Estrogen is necessary for the development of female characteristics, is essential for childbearing, and is involved in cholesterol regulation and in maintaining proper bone density. Phytoestrogens can produce a similar biological response. For this reason, phytoestrogens have been studied as therapeutic agents in treating breast cancer, prostate cancer, osteoporosis, menopausal symptoms, and reducing the risk of heart disease.

Normally the amounts of these chemicals in plants are very small and have little effect on us. However, if we consume a large amount of

116

foods rich in phytoestrogens over an extended period of time, they can have a significant physiological effect.

The most prominent plant hormones are the growth factors. There are three major classes of plant growth hormones—auxins, gibberellins, and cytokinins. Plant growth hormones were first discovered in the late 1800s. Japanese farmers observed that their rice grew very tall when it was infected by a fungal disease called Bakanae disease or "foolish seedling." This fungus was later given the name *Gibberella fujikuroi*. Scientists eventually identified the group of compounds in the fungus that stimulated growth in the rice and named them *gibberellins*. Gibberellins, and later auxins, were identified in many plants. Cytokinins were the last to be identified.

Growth is accomplished in two ways—cell division and cell enlargement. Increase in cell number by division does not in itself result in growth—an increase in size of the divided cells is also needed. In general, auxins and gibberellins promote cell enlargement while cytokinins promote cell division. These hormones produce a wide variety of effects and interact with each other and the environment in such complex ways that their actions are still not fully understood.

Growth hormones are produced in actively growing tissues such as roots, shoot apex, young leaves, and seeds. Growth hormones are particularly important in seeds because from here embryonic cells multiply, differentiate, and grow into adult plants. While all three types of hormones are important for plant growth and development, it is the cytokinins that are of greatest importance to us.

COCONUT CYTOKININS

Plant cytokinins are not to be confused with *cytokines* which are produced in the human body. Cytokines are hormone-like substances that are produced by white blood cells. They are involved in reproduction, growth and development, homeostatic regulation, healing and repair, blood clotting, and immunity. The similarity in the names is not a coincidence. Both hormones have somewhat similar duties in their own respective spheres. Cytokinins are the plant version of cytokines. We will talk more about cytokines later. The spellings of these two words are so similar they can easily be confused. Take a minute to remember the different endings so that you can distinguish which is which later on; cytokin**ins** for plants and cytokin**es** for humans.

Coconut water is important in modern botanical science because it was the key that led to the discovery of cytokinins and to a greater understanding of plant growth and differentiation.

In the 1930s and 1940s researchers knew that plants could regenerate themselves. Stem and leaf cuttings could form roots and develop into entire plants. But how they did this was a mystery. To understand this effect, botanists studied cell cultures under controlled conditions in the laboratory. Tissue cultures, however, either would not grow or grew only for a limited time. Getting a whole plant to develop from a culture was elusive.

Researchers knew the importance of vitamins and minerals in the medium culture and tried various combinations. The big breakthrough came in 1941 when Johannes Van Overbeek and colleagues discovered that adding coconut water to the medium greatly stimulated cell growth.[1] Working with young carrot embryos Van Overbeek cultured them in the coconut water and then planted them in soil. Like magic, the embryos sprang to life and began to grow rapidly. In four days the embryos increased in volume by over 300 times. In 10 days they increased in volume by 8,000 times. In comparison, the controls showed no growth. For the first time, cultured cells developed into normal adult plants. Van Overbeek's studies demonstrated that plant cells carry the DNA to produce an entire plant. All that is needed are the nutrients and plant growth hormones.

Van Overbeek recognized that coconut water provided the missing growth factors necessary for the plant to grow and mature. He and other researchers at the time referred to coconut water as coconut "milk," which is a common misnomer even today. In their published studies, the term "coconut milk" actually refers to coconut water.

Coconut water contains all the nutrients needed, including growth factors, for a plant cutting to grow, differentiate, and develop fully. For this reason, it soon became the standard for use in culture studies. Coconut water also found use as a growth enhancer, sort of like a fertilizer supplement, in nurseries and plant studies. In many cases it increases vegetable growth, yield, and vitamin content. Vegetables treated with coconut water have significantly higher vitamin A (beta-carotene), B-6, and C as well as chlorophyll content.[2]

The search to identify the specific growth factors in coconut water led to the discovery of cytokinins. The first cytokinin wasn't isolated and identified until 1955. The name given to this compound was *kinetin* because of its ability to promote cytokinesis (cell division). The term cytokinin has come to be used to describe all plant hormones with kinetin-like growth promoting activity.

Ironically, the discovery of kinetin did not come from coconut or from any other plant, but from a fish. It was found in the DNA of herring sperm.[3] While researchers were trying to identify the growth factors in coconut water, by chance they discovered that herring sperm also stimulated plant growth just as coconut water did. This led them to investigate further and finally to the discovery of kinetin.

The first plant derived cytokinin wasn't identified until 1961. It was called zeatin and was very similar to kinetin in form and function. Since that time many natural and synthetic plant growth hormones have been identified. Although kinetin was initially discovered in fish sperm, it was later found in plants. All of the cytokinins have similar chemical structure and growth regulating effects.

Plants contain a mixture of all three classes of growth hormones (auxins, gibberellins, and cytokinins). The concentration of the various hormones varies within plants. Seeds are especially rich in cytokinins because they are essential for the rapid growth and differentiation of the developing seedling. Coconut, which is the largest seed in existence, contains the highest amount of cytokinins of any plant. Therefore, coconut water is a very rich source of these plant hormones. Coconut contains at least nine different cytokinins, including kinetin.[4-5] It also contains a variety of other growth regulators such as gibberellins, auxins, ethylene, and abscissic acid. This is why it is so successful in stimulating and regulating growth in tissue cultures.

Seeds contain tissue known as endosperm. This material is essential for the survival and development of the seedling. Endosperm is the starchy, nutrient-rich substance found in seeds, grains, and nuts. It provides the plant embryo with the nutrients and hormones it needs to develop into a growing plant. The endosperm essentially provides the

Coconuts can remain alive for several months after they have matured and fallen to the ground. They often float in the ocean for long periods of time before coming to rest on shore where they sprout and grow. The living tissue inside the hard dense shell is hermetically sealed, 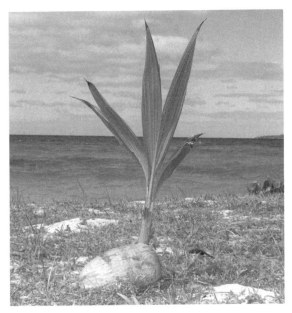 thus keeping out sea water, bacteria, mold, and toxins. The husk also provides a layer of protection, primarily against trauma resulting from falling out of the tree and the pounding of the ocean waves.

food the seedling needs until roots, stem, and leaves have developed sufficiently to sustain continued growth and development.

Coconut water is liquid endosperm. Coconut meat is solid endosperm. As the coconut matures the water is transformed into the meat. A coconut seedling can survive for nearly 12 months on just the liquid and solid endosperm, which gives plenty of time for a wandering coconut to travel on the ocean, find a home, and take root.

Endosperm is the food that nourishes infant seedlings. It is analogous to the milk mammals feed their young for the first few months of life, until weaning. Coconut water, being liquid endosperm, is in essence the "milk" consumed by the coconut seedling. This may explain part of the reason why coconut water has often been termed coconut milk. However, coconut milk is technically the juice extracted from coconut meat and is not the same as coconut water.

PLANT HORMONES AND HUMAN HEALTH
The Anti-Aging Hormone

The search for the fountain of youth has been going on for thousands of years. Even today scientists continue the search using modern scientific methods. Several compounds in nature have been found that seem to promote youth or at least slow down various aspects of aging. Cytokinins have shown to be some of the most promising of these compounds. Their anti-aging effects on plants are well known. Interestingly, these plant hormones appear to have a positive influence on animal and human tissues as well.

One of the ways cytokinins retard the effects of aging is by blocking one of the major factors involved in the aging processes—free radicals.[6] Cytokinins are potent antioxidants that stop the destructive action of free radicals. Free radicals are renegade molecules that damage proteins, fats, and DNA. A lifetime of exposure to free radicals brings about many of the degenerative conditions associated with aging. Those people (as well as plants and animals) who experience the greatest exposure to free radicals generally show symptoms of aging the soonest.

Both plants and humans are continuously exposed to the destructive action of free radicals. The brown aging spots (i.e., lipofuscin) that often appear on the skin as we age are caused by the free-radical induced destruction of proteins and fats in our skin. Damage to structural proteins and fats can lead to loss of function; for example, damage to collagen in the skin causes wrinkles and sagging—obvious sings of aging. Collagen damage in blood vessel walls can lead to vessel wall stiffness and hypertension, and to the formation of atherosclerosis (arterial plaque). Similar processes in the kidneys, liver, and other organs can lead to the decreased performance of these organs. Neurological degeneration, such as senility and Alzheimer's disease, is caused by the destructive action of free radicals.

Free radicals attack on a cellular level. They damage cell walls in plants and cell membranes in animals and cell organelles, including the mitochondria that produce energy and the nuclei which house DNA. When DNA is damaged by free radicals, it can cause mutations that kill the cell or cause it to become cancerous.

Free radicals are continually being formed in our environment and in our bodies. They can be caused by a number of things including radiation (including UV radiation from the sun), physical stress, illness, and various chemicals in our food and environment. They even occur as a part of the normal processes of metabolism. Fortunately, antioxidant nutrients and enzymes in our bodies arrest free radicals, tempering their destructive potential. The effects of aging are accelerated when people are exposed to high levels of free radicals or have low levels of antioxidants. Antioxidant status is determined primarily by diet. Vitamins A, C, D, and E, zinc, selenium, and other nutrients act as antioxidants or are incorporated into antioxidant enzymes synthesized in the body. That is one of the reasons why good nutrition is so important to health and why a diet rich in fresh fruits and vegetables has repeatedly been shown to help prevent degenerative diseases.

Eating foods rich in antioxidants is one way we can help block the destructive effects of free radicals. Part of the reason for the anti-aging effects of cytokinins is due to their antioxidant properties.[7] When applied to human skin kinetin has shown to exhibit greater antioxidant protection against UV radiation than many other antioxidants such as vitamin C, CoQ10, and alpha lipoic acid.[8]

While the antioxidant properties of cytokinins are important and helpful, they are not the primary means by which aging is affected. One of the primary functions of cytokinins is to regulate cell division. They also influence the rate at which plants age. Depending on the amount of cytokinins present, the aging process in plants can be either accelerated or retarded. One of the active sites of cytokinin production is in the roots. From here the hormone is carried by the sap throughout the plant—much like our bloodstream disperses hormones. Portions of plants that are deprived of a continuous supply of cytokinins age faster than normal. Conversely, if additional cytokinins are added to a plant, normal aging is retarded.

When plant stems are separated from the roots, cytokinin is no longer delivered to the rest of the plant. Putting a plant in a vase of water keeps it from immediately drying out, but because there is no longer a source of cytokinins, the plant soon withers and dies. If, however, cytokinins are added to the water , the plant will stay alive much longer. The processes that cause the plant to whiter and die are slowed down.*

The anti-aging effects of cytokinins in living plants are now well established. The next question researchers wanted an answer to was if cytokinins had a similar effect on other living organisms? Apparently they do. Animal tissue, like that of a plant, when surgically removed ages very fast. Preserving living tissue for culture studies or transplantation is important to researchers and physicians. In order to ensure tissue quality at a later time they are stored in special solutions that retard aging. Coconut water has been shown to be effective in prolonging the life of animal tissues. In fact, it is even more effective than Braun-Collins solutions that have been formulated for this purpose.[9]

Cytokinins have been shown to retard aging in human tissue as well. Normal human cells, as they age, go through a progressive and irreversible accumulation of changes until they reach a stage at which they finally die. Young cells are plump, round, and smooth. As they age they become irregular in shape, flatten out, enlarge, and fill up with debris; cell division slows down and eventually stops, which is ultimately followed by death.

When cytokinins are added to the culture medium, cells don't act their age. The normal sequence of aging slows down considerably. Cells do not undergo the severe degenerative changes that ordinarily occur.[10-11] Although the total lifespan of human cells is not affected much, the cells remain significantly more youthful and functional throughout their lifetime. For example, treated cells after they have reached the final stage of their lifespan and no longer divide, look and function like untreated cells half their age. Treated cells never undergo the severe degenerative changes experienced by untreated cells. In all respects, their youth is extended into old age.

One of the signs of aging is the increase in protein content of cells. This occurs as a result of incomplete division of the cell's contents during mitosis (cell division). Cells tend to accumulate residual debris and often end up with multiple nuclei that have not properly separated. Cytokinins help regulate cell division so that there is almost a complete absence of cell debris even into old age.

---

*Adding coconut water to a vase of water will not necessarily increase the life of a plant. The reason for this is because coconut water is such a good medium for growth that bacteria flourish, which adversely affects the life of the plant.

What happens in cell cultures may not always reflect what happens in living organisms. It's important that the studies performed in cell cultures be supported by studies on living organisms. Such studies are showing that cytokinins do have a similar effect on animals and humans.

An interesting study was done using fruit flies. Fruit flies are popular in aging studies because their lifespan is measured in days rather than years. This allows researchers to evaluate aging parameters in a relatively short amount of time.

The average lifespan of the fruit fly is only 35 days. Even long-lived fruit flies don't last more than 70 or 75 days. Low levels of kinetin added to the diet of fruit flies raises the median lifespan to over 50 days with the oldest surviving for over 90 days.[12] If we translate these figures in terms of human lifespan, it would equate to an average increase of at least 16 years.

Feeding fruit flies kinetin has dramatic effects on their development, aging, and longevity. The researchers involved in these studies state: "The life-prolonging effects of kinetin are not merely due to a slowing down of the developmental stages, but are mainly due to the reduction in age-specific death rates and slowing down of aging. This suggests the kinetin prevents early deaths either by maintaining the efficiency of various repair and defense systems or by reducing the accumulation of metabolic defects and debris that may have harmful effects on cellular physiology and biochemistry."

Kinetin is the most commonly used cytokinin in aging studies. Because of kinetin's anti-aging effects on plant, animal, and human cells, it has been tested as a topical ointment for the possible treatment for aging spots, wrinkles, sagging, and dry or rough skin. One of the factors that causes wrinkles and sagging skin is the aging and breakdown of connective tissues in the skin. Connective tissues give the skin strength and elasticity. When kinetin is applied to the skin, it stimulates cell division of connective tissue which replaces older, damaged tissue with functionally younger tissue.[13] The result is that on the surface of the skin, wrinkles and sagging tend to flatten out and firm up. Dry, aging skin is replaced with smoother, softer skin.

Topical solutions containing kinetin have also been shown to reduce or normalize abnormal pigmentation such as aging spots.[14] In studies using human subjects lasting up to 100 days, no adverse effects have been reported and, therefore, kinetin is considered safe to use for long-term application. As a result of these studies, some facial creams and lotions on the market contain kinetin as one of the active ingredients.

Although kinetin may reverse some of the age-related changes in human tissues, its effects are most pronounced in preventing or retarding age-related changes. Most importantly, treatment of human cells with kinetin did not cause premature cell death (a sign of toxicity) nor did it induce extra cell proliferation which is a sign of potential carcinogenesis. In this respect, kinetin differs significantly from other so-called anti-aging compounds which can either cause some cell death (for example, retinol) or can promote cell proliferation (for example, serum growth factors and carnosine).

While most of these anti-aging studies have focused on kinetin, all of the cytokinins seem to work together synergistically in producing their anti-aging effects.[15] While cell division and antioxidant effects of cytokinins are involved in the anti-aging process, the exact mechanisms of action are not yet fully known. Some evidence indicates that cytokinins are involved in signal transduction which may stimulate other defense pathways, such as DNA repair.

It is believed that what cytokinins do when added to cell cultures and when applied to the skin, they can also do inside the body as well. Therefore consuming a good source of cytokinins may have a rejuvenating or anti-aging effect systemically. Investigators theorize that because of cytokinins' antioxidant and anti-aging properties, they may have potential in the prevention and treatment of medical conditions such as cancer, heart disease, cataract, macular degeneration, and Alzheimer's disease. The regular consumption of coconut water may prove beneficial in preventing some of these conditions.

The Anti-Cancer Hormone

Since cytokinins are *growth* hormones and stimulate cell division one might ask: is it possible that they may over-stimulate growth to the point that cells become cancerous? Actually the opposite is true. Research as far back as the 1960s shows that when cytokinins are added to cancerous tissue, abnormal growth is retarded.[16]

Much of the early research on cytokinins was funded by The American Cancer Society. Because of their similarity to human cytokines, which have anti-cancer effects, researchers theorized that plant cytokinins might also be useful in the fight against cancer. Subsequently, cytokinins have been reported to have anti-cancer effects in human and animal cells.[17-22]

While cytokinins do stimulate cell division, they do not significantly increase the lifespan of cells or the total number of cell divisions. This lack of stimulation of cell proliferation is an extremely interesting characteristic which distinguishes cytokinins from other compounds which affect proliferative capacity of human cells in culture. Therefore, cytokinins can delay the onset of many aging characteristics without forcing the cells to undergo additional proliferation.

Every cell in our bodies came from a single cell. As we were developing in the womb, cells differentiated, some becoming bone cells, others skin cells, or blood cells, and so forth. Each cell has a specific purpose and function. Every cell carries the same genetic code but functions in different capacities. This differentiation is essential for the growth, survival, and propagation of the body. A mass of similar cells or cells that have no specific function would be useless.

One of the characteristics of cancer is undifferentiation. When cells become cancerous, they lose their unique functional capacities. Liver cells, for instance, that have become cancerous no longer function as liver cells. In essence, they become parasites, serving no useful purpose, yet consuming vital nutrients. Cancerous cells grow rapidly and, unlike normal cells, don't have a finite lifespan. They can continue to divide and multiply indefinitely. As tumors grow, they interfere with the function of other organs and tissues. If interference becomes severe enough, it can cause death.

In addition to regulating cell division, cytokinins also regulate cell differentiation. In other words, they encourage undifferiented cells to develop into specific types of cells with a useful purpose. In plants, cytokinins induce callus (clusters of undifferentiated plant cells that grow over wounds) to redifferentiate into buds. Because of similarities in cancer and callus cells, researchers have examined the effect cytokinins have in promoting differentiation in human tissues. Like with plants, cytokinins induce changes in cancer cells that cause differentiation.[23-25]

Studies show cytokinins are also effective at inducing apoptosis or programmed cell death in cancer cells.[26-27] Apoptosis, a natural process, is important because it limits the lifespan of cells. When cells get old, they die. This is how it is supposed to work. Cells are programmed to self-destruct after a certain amount of time. This way, new cells replace the old. Cancer cells are diseased and have lost the program information that limits their lifespan. Cancer cells, if given adequate nourishment, can live virtually forever, continually multiplying and growing. One of the areas of cancer research is reactivating apoptosis so that cancer cells die and are removed like ordinary cells.

Another way cytokinins help to protect against cancer is through their antioxidant properties. Antioxidants protect against free-radical damage that can cause cancerous mutations to DNA.[28] Cytokinins are proven to have anti-cancer effects and when included in the diet may be helpful in cancer prevention.

Cytokinins Help Prevent Heart Disease

Cytokinins have been shown to help protect the heart and arteries from conditions that promote heart disease. This is intriguing because it suggests a way to help fight the world's number one killer.

Oxidation, caused by free radicals, is one of the primary mechanisms that damages artery walls, causes inflammation, and promotes cholesterol accumulation and the formation of arterial plaque. As plaque builds up inside artery walls, the flow of blood becomes restricted. Every tissue and organ in the body demands a continuous supply of oxygen from the blood in order to live. If we were denied oxygen for just a short amount of time, we would suffocate and die. Likewise, tissues and organs rely on a continuous supply of oxygen to maintain life. Cut off blood circulation, and you prevent the delivery of life-giving oxygen; consequently, cells and tissues began to suffocate. This is exactly what happens when a person suffers a heart attack or a stroke. Antioxidants help fight heart disease by stopping the destructive action of free radicals. As potent antioxidants, cytokinins help to keep arteries open and plaque free.

One of the primary risk factors for heart disease is high blood pressure. As blood pressure increases, the force exerted against artery walls increases. This puts more stress on the artery wall which can cause inflammation and minute injuries. These injuries set into motion the processes by which scar tissue, blood clots, fat, and cholesterol accumulate to form plaque.

One of the things that increases blood pressure is blood stickiness. Blood contains special proteins known as platelets. At the site of an injury, these platelets are activated and become sticky and cause blood cells to clump together and form clots. Clotting is necessary to stop bleeding and facilitate tissue repair. Unwanted clotting, however, is a problem.

High blood pressure can initiate injury to artery walls. These injuries signal platelets to become sticky, which thickens the blood and causes blood pressure to increase. As blood pressure increases, artery walls are further damaged, thus perpetuating the entire process, making the situation worse. Doctors often prescribe blood thinning medications to reduce blood stickiness and lower blood pressure.

Cytokinins are natural blood thinners and can be helpful in keeping blood pressure under control.[29] One of the major causes of heart attacks and strokes is getting a blood clot lodged in an artery. Blood clots often form on the inside surface of damaged arteries. If one of these clots happens to break loose, it can travel toward the heart or brain where it may become lodged in an artery already narrowed by plaque. Acting as a plug, it stops the flow of oxygenated blood, thus causing a heart attack or stroke. Cytokinins help to keep unwanted clots from forming, thus reducing the risk of experiencing a heart attack or stroke.

Thromboxane A2 is a hormone-like substance produced by platelets that causes blood clotting and the constriction of blood vessels. Sticky blood in narrowed arteries makes it more difficult for blood to flow, which increases blood pressure. Thromboxane is named for its role in clot formation (thrombosis). Cytokinins significantly inhibit thromboxane A2 formation and are so effective at reducing platelet aggregation that they are being investigated as a potential therapeutic agent for preventing arterial thrombosis.[30]

Reducing blood stickiness, lowering high blood pressure, and protecting arteries from injuries that lead to plaque formation are some of the things researchers are discovering in relation to cytokinins. As research continues, it is likely that investigators will discover additional benefits directly related to heart health.

It is well known that diet affects the health of our heart and circulatory system. As a part of the diet, cytokinins may play a role in protecting us from heart disease. The foods with the highest cytokinin content are nuts and seeds, with coconut being by far the best source. Studies indicate that nuts and seeds do reduce heart disease risk. Researchers at Penn State University reviewed the data from 16 previously published studies. Their goal was to examine the effect nuts have on heart health. What they discovered was that nut consumption reduces heart disease risk. Eating an ounce of nuts five or more times a week reduces risk of heart disease by up to 39 percent.[31] An ounce of nuts is about 3-4 tablespoons. That's not much.

The types of nuts included almonds, Brazil nuts, cashews, hazelnuts, macadamia nuts, pecans, pistachios, walnuts, and peanuts. Technically, peanuts are not nuts, they are legumes. However, all are seeds rich in cytokinins.

The investigators were not able to determine if any specific type of nut was better than any other because of limitations in the data. The nutrients in the nuts were quite variable and the researchers could not identify any particular substance that was of greatest importance. They attributed the heart protective effect to a synergistic combination of protein, fiber, fat, vitamins, minerals, and phytochemicals (this would include plant hormones). In other words, they really had no idea what gives nuts their protective effect.

Two earlier studies—the Nurses' Health Study[32] and the Adventist Health Study[33]—assessed the diets of over 110,000 men and women in relation to coronary heart disease. These researchers linked the intake of five 1-ounce servings per week to a 35-50 percent reduction in heart disease incidence and death. This is actual reduction in incidence of heart disease and not just an assessment of risk. Again, the reason why nuts were protective was not determined.

From what we know about cytokinins, it is possible that they are responsible, or at least partially responsible, for the protective effect seen in these studies. Coconut meat and coconut water being the highest dietary sources of cytokinins, would offer the greatest amount of protection.

Judging from population studies, this seems to be the case. Populations with the highest coconut consumption have the lowest heart disease rates in the world.[34] For instance, studies with coconut eating populations in Papua New Guinea show a complete absence of heart disease and stroke. Even the oldest members of the population who are in their upper 90s show no signs of clogging in their arteries.[35] This same absence of heart disease is found in coconut eating populations around the world.

The American Heart Association gathers statistics on heart disease deaths from many countries. In a recent listing of heart disease deaths from 35 countries those with the highest rates were in Eastern Europe followed by a mixture from Western Europe, Latin America, North America, and Asia. The country on the list with the lowest death rate from heart disease was Japan, at 548 deaths per 100,000 population. This was less than a third of the highest rate reported which was Russia at 1802 per 100,000. None of the countries on the list were major coconut consumers. Even the Japanese don't eat much coconut, but in the Philippines they do. Data from the Philippines wasn't included in the original list because it wasn't available at the time the list was compiled. However, information from the Philippines shows a heart disease death rate of only 120 per 100,000. This is even lower than Japan's. In fact, the heart disease death rate in the Philippines is less than a fourth of that of Japan![36]

Even within the Philippines, where coconut consumption is the highest, heart disease is the lowest. The Bicol region of the Philippines has the highest intake of coconut because they cook most of their food in coconut milk. The Bicolanos have the lowest incidence of heart disease in the country.

As traditional coconut eating populations around the world become more globalized, consumption of western foods has been increasing. Unfortunately, coconut is being displaced in the diet with white bread, chips, cookies, soda, and other packaged, convenience foods. Consequently, heart disease rates are rising in places where it was relatively rare before.

Wound Healing

We often marvel at how indestructible children are. They are full of energy and can play hard all day without seeming to tire. They fall, get hurt, and in no time at all, evidence of any injury is gone. Don't we all wish we had the recuperative power of our youth? As we age, many of the biological processes in our bodies slow down or become less efficient. One of these processes is the ability to repair and recover from injuries. Wounds, for instance, take longer to heal. One of the reasons for this is that cytokine production at injured sites becomes less efficient as we age. However, if cytokines are applied topically to the injury, healing is accelerated. In studies with aged rats, a single topical application of cytokines to wounds increases the rate of healing to match that experienced by young rats.[37]

In animals and humans, cytokines are essential in the healing of wounds and injuries. In plants, cytokinins are also necessary for the healing process. Cytokinins are needed to trigger cell division and new tissue growth. When plants are injured, they go through a healing process similar to ours. New tissue called a callus forms over the injury. For instance, when a limb on a tree is cut off, a callus is formed over the injury. In time, the cut is completely healed over.

Since cytokinins have been shown to stimulate cell division and repair in human tissue as well as plant tissue, they may be useful in treating injuries. One of the traditional therapeutic uses for coconut water is to speed the healing of wounds and boils when applied topically. Taking this idea one step further, when consumed it may be possible for cytokinins to produce a healing effect within the digestive tract. This offers a potential therapeutic effect for a number of digestive disorders where tissues along the gastrointestinal tract are damaged, including ulcers, ulcerative colitis, Crohn's disease, celiac disease, leaky gut syndrome, among others. People with these conditions often gain substantial relief simply by adding coconut into their daily diet. Coconut meat as well as the water contains cytokinins.

In a health column published by King Features Syndicate a reader writes: "More than 20 years ago I was diagnosed with irritable bowel syndrome (IBS). Tests revealed no cause. Diarrhea attacks accompanied by severe abdominal pain rarely gave me time to find a bathroom before it was too late. I would suffer several times a week. At 6 feet 2 inches tall I weighted only 147 pounds and could not gain weight, even eating 5,000 calories a day. Imodium A-D daily provided minimal help. Ten months ago I read in your column about a man with Crohn's disease who had been helped by eating two Archway Coconut Macaroons daily. I had nothing to lose, so I gave it a try. IT HAS

CHANGED MY LIFE! In those past 10 months I have had only a few mild attacks, none involving pain. Even the worst of these was milder than a good day before. I stopped carrying a change of clothes in my car, as I haven't needed them once. Twenty years of suffering, and all I needed to do was eat cookies! There is not one medication on the market that can boast fewer side effects. My weight is now stable at 180 pounds, ideal for my height."

Teresa Graedon, Ph.D., the co-author of *The People's Pharmacy Guide to Herbal and Home Remedies*, says that during the research for her book she heard enough testimonials about the benefit of using coconut for Crohn's disease that she was convinced that this is one home remedy that may have important medical significance and believes strongly that more research should be pursued in this area.

Hair Growth

Everybody likes a full head of hair. For those who are a little shy on top, the idea of a tonic that can restore a youthful head of hair is enticing. Drugs have been developed that can help stop hair loss or even restore growth in some cases. But many people don't like taking drugs, don't like the side effects, or just don't respond to treatment. A natural, harmless, topical ointment may be just around the corner.

According to dermatologist Vermen Verallo-Rowell, M.D. coconut water may be useful as a natural hair tonic and hair restorer. While studying the effects of coconut oil as a skin moisturizer, antioxidant, and disinfectant, she discovered that coconut water has the potential to revive hair growth.[38]

Hair grows in stages. There is an active period of growth that lasts for about 2-3 years. During this time hair grows at a rate of about 6 inches (15 cm) a year. The hair then goes into a transition stage for 2-3 weeks before entering a dormant stage that lasts about 3 months. No growth occurs in the last two stages and during the dormant stage, hair falls out. New hairs take their place, and the process repeats itself. Normally, up to 90 percent of the hair is actively growing while 10-15 percent is falling out. We lose about 50-100 hairs a day.

The amount of time hair remains in the growing phase is genetically determined and changes over time. When we are young, it may remain in this phase for 6-7 years. As we age, this period of growth shortens.

Thus, we all experience some thinning as we grow older. Hormones also affect hair growth, which accounts for some men being bald.

If you are genetically programmed to become bald, a signal is sent that slows down cytokine production in the hair follicles on the top of the head. Consequently, over time the follicles gradually grow smaller and the hairs they produce become finer until they are too small to be seen and the head looks bald. Lower down on the scalp and face cytokines continue to stimulate normal hair growth.

Dr. Verallo-Rowell theorizes that cytokinins may be able to stop hair loss and even restore hair to a balding head. Since cytokinins, like cytokines, can stimulate growth in human cells, they may be useful in stimulating hair follicles to grow as well. This growth would produce thicker strands of hair, which could possibly bring back a full head of hair. She suggests that applying coconut water regularly to the scalp may provide enough cytokinins to stimulate hair growth. For this therapy to work, a person would need to massage the water into the scalp daily over an extended period of time to see any changes. At this point, this is just a theory, but Dr. Verallo-Rowell is actively doing research in this area.

DISCOVERING THE BENEFITS OF COCONUT WATER

Those people who live among coconut trees and consume coconut water daily have discovered many of the coconut's health giving properties, not all of which are discussed at length in this book. Some of the effects, such as an increase in libido, are believed to be more potent with the use of fresh coconut water. As the water ages, it is thought to lose some of its potency. But for oral rehydration commercially packaged coconut water appears to be just as effective as fresh. The vitamins, minerals, growth hormones, and other substances are present in both fresh and packaged coconut water.

The coconut growth hormones are particularly hearty. They can remain active and viable even when exposed to heat, acids, or fermentation.[39] Even when coconuts are put into storage for long periods of time, the hormone levels do not fall. In fact, they increase! As coconuts age, whether they are growing on a tree or not, hormone levels increase. So the whole coconuts you get at the store, which

Coconut Water Cured My PMS!

Moodiness, bloating, cramps. We all know what that means—PMS! And for some women, it's so awful, it turns life upside down. Just ask 30-year-old Katie Davis. As a teenager, the drug Midol was all Katie needed to handle her periods. But by her 20s she had developed full-blown PMS. Starting a week before her period, she had mood swings so severe, a TV commercial could reduce her to tears; fatigue so extreme, no amount of sleep made her feel rested; plus, headaches, cramps, even irritable bowel syndrome.

It got so bad that Katie had to tell her boss about her problems to avoid getting fired—because when her period started, she was in so much pain, she'd have to call in sick two days every month! Desperate, she tried everything from heat packs to birth control pills. But nothing helped.

Then, she confided in her friend Karen. "I'm sick of spending half my life feeling sick and crazy!"

"You should try coconut water," Karen suggested. "I've heard it works wonders on female problems!"

"Coconut water?" Katie wondered. Where do I even buy it? But a conversation at her local health-food store answered all her questions.

"Coconut water is made out of the fluid in coconuts," they explained. "It has high levels of potassium and magnesium plus vitamin C and trace amounts of copper, phosphorus, and sulfur, so it corrects electrolyte imbalances. Nutritionists call it 'Nature's Gatorade.' It's even recommended by the World Health Organization for stomach problems."

So Katie tried it and was pleasantly surprised. It tasted good. But would it work? Drinking a 12-ounce bottle three

Continued on next page.

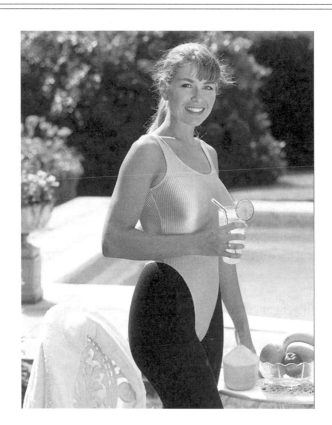

times a week, Katie soon noticed little changes—like feeling less tired after a workout.

Then, a few weeks later, "This is incredible!" Katie marveled. For the first time since she was 17, she breezed through her period without mood swings, cramps, or mad dashes to the bathroom. Today, Katie drinks coconut water before and during every period—and swears by it! "It feels great not having to look at the calendar to know what kind of day I'm going to have," Katie says. "Thanks to coconut water, all my days are good!"

Adapted from: Capetta, A. *Woman's World*. February 2007.

were picked one or two months earlier, contain more growth hormones than when they were freshly picked. Coconuts continue to live even after they have been removed from the tree. Like any seed, they can germinate and grow months after leaving the tree. Young coconuts that have been stored for over three months continue their lifecycle. The water even continues to be converted into coconut meat as if it were still attached to the tree.

As you have seen in this chapter, cytokinins in coconut water possess well defined anti-aging properties. They retard aging in plants and in human cells in culture, and slow down the aging and prolong the lifespan of insects. Topical application of lotions containing cytokinins have shown to reduce aging pigmentation, wrinkles, sagging, and improve skin texture. Cytokinins are effective free radical scavengers and block many of the detrimental effects of oxidation, including the breakdown of collagen in human tissues. They protect against many of the conditions that promote heart disease and atherosclerosis, the most common cause of death. They protect cells from the processes that promote cancer, and they trigger cancerous cells to self-destruct. They promote healing and the formation of new tissue and may be useful in preventing hair loss or restoring hair. Coconut water is the richest natural dietary source of these health promoting cytokinins. In this respect, coconut water can be considered a fountain of youth.

In a recent survey of all published studies on kinetin—the most studied of the cytokinins—European researchers acknowledged the potential of young coconut water stating, "Its presence in young coconut coupled with the anti-aging activity suggests the benefits of drinking coconut water as a healthy beverage should be further explored."[40] There is no doubt that as further research involving coconut water is done, we will discover many new and exciting health benefits to this remarkable beverage.

Gastrointestinal Health

A GUT FEELING

When Jordan Rubin headed off to Florida State University to begin his freshman year, he had no idea that his life was about to change. He joined the cheerleading squad, was active in sports and campus life, and worked hard to maintain good grades. When he returned home for the summer, he began to experience periodic feelings of extreme exhaustion punctuated by onslaughts of nausea, stomach cramps, painful mouth sores, and diarrhea.

He went to the doctor who tested him for various viral infections, but the tests were all negative. So the doctor prescribed antibiotics and sent him home. When the new school year started, his problems grew worse. Endless trips to the bathroom and lack of energy forced him to drop out of the cheerleading squad and curtail other activities. His once muscular 180 pound frame shrank to 145. He struggled to attend class.

He started taking dietary supplements and experimented with different diets, but nothing seemed to work. Every decision he made hinged on the location of the nearest bathroom. Finally, suffering from a high fever, he went to the hospital. He stayed for two weeks. During this time doctors examined him carefully. Their diagnoses? Crohn's disease—chronic inflammation and ulceration along the digestive tract.

His future looked bleak. There was little the physicians could do for him. Medications would help relieve some of the pain and discomfort, but the disease usually progresses with increasing severity and the need for more medications and perhaps surgery. Even with medications, his condition failed to improve. He rushed to the toilet up to 30 times daily—day and night. He says, "I can only describe my situation as experiencing the pain of a 24 hour stomach virus or a bad case of food poisoning day and night for two years." His weight dropped to 104 pounds. He became so emaciated that he looked like a concentration camp victim. His doctor recommended that they surgically remove his colon and part of his small intestine. He refused. This was something he wasn't ready to do.

Desperately searching for an answer he tried multiple remedies without success. During his research he learned about the workings of the digestive tract and importance of balancing the environment within. He discovered that the longest living populations in the world consumed "live" foods that abound with nutrients, enzymes, and beneficial microorganisms. They did not eat "lifeless," commercially processed food loaded with sugar, preservatives, and other additives. He began to change the way he ate. He began eating whole, organic foods. His diet included kefir (a fermented milk), raw sauerkraut (fermented cabbage), organic juices, and lots of fresh fruits and vegetables. He also added a dietary supplement containing homeostatic soil organisms—soil bacteria.

The dietary changes worked their magic. Within 45 days he regained 29 pounds, a clear sign he was improving. It took time to overcome years of illness, and two years later, on his 21st birthday he celebrated his complete recovery.

The reason for Jordan's illness was that his internal environment was out of balance. As long as he remained out of balance, he couldn't get better. It was only after he made efforts to correct the problem that he was able to get better. A key factor in his recovery was the consumption of probiotics—friendly gut bacteria. These good bacteria, along with healthful foods, reestablished harmony in his digestive tract.

Digestive problems are epidemic nowadays—heartburn, constipation, bloating, indigestion, ulcers, etc. Most of us ignore the symptoms, attributing them to simply poor digestion or spicy foods. The real problem is an imbalance in the body's inner ecology.

It has been said that the key to good health lies within the gut. If there is a problem with digestive function, it will affect the health and well-being of the entire body. Balancing our inner ecology then is of prime importance in achieving and maintaining good health.

INNER ECOLOGY

A community of organisms within a specific environment or habitat is called an ecosystem. In a forest, for instance, it consists of specific species of trees, bushes, grasses, animals, insects, and microorganisms, all of which live in harmonious balance with each other. The plant and animal life in each ecosystem is governed in large measure by the environment. The wildlife you see in a rainforest is different from what you find in a desert or on a mountain peak. But in every case, there is a balance in which all things live in equilibrium with each other. As long as nothing disrupts the ecosystem, it will continue indefinitely.

Our bodies have their own ecosystem teeming with microscopic organisms. For the most part, we live in harmony with them. The human body is home to more than 400 species of microorganisms, mostly bacteria and fungi, collectively known as microflora. The greatest population of microflora lives within our digestive tract. In fact, each of us carries around about 3.5 pounds of these organisms inside our intestines. Most of these microflora are not harmful, and in fact, many are vital to our health. These good organisms, primarily bacteria, are called probiotics.

In addition to friendly bacteria, we also carry around unfriendly organisms. These are opportunistic organisms that will cause disease or discomfort whenever given the opportunity. Like any ecosystem in nature, there are those inhabitants that can cause problems for everyone else. When the ecosystem is in balance, however, these troublemakers are kept under control and do not pose much of a threat.

For example, in your backyard, aphids may infect your trees. Aphids are tiny parasitic insects that suck the juices from plants. These tiny insects cause the leaves to curl up, turn brown, and die, preventing the tree from producing energy from the sun. If allowed to multiply and spread, aphids can overwhelm and kill an entire tree. Even though the tree stands tall and appears invincible, it can be downed by an insect the size of a pinhead. Fortunately, the ecology is kept in balance by other creatures. In this case, the ladybug. Ladybugs feed on aphids. As long as there are plenty of ladybugs around aphids don't cause too much problem. Everything is in harmony.

Our digestive tract is like your backyard. Friendly bacteria, like ladybugs, keep unfriendly organisms from getting out of hand. Everything is in balance. Your digestion is good and your health is good, just as nature intended. However, if something were to happen to the good bacteria, it could cause serious consequences.

For instance, let's say beetles were attacking some of your shrubs so you spray your backyard with a pesticide. The pesticide not only poisons and kills the beetles but also the ladybugs (which also happen to be beetles). Without ladybugs, aphids seize the opportunity to multiply out of control, causing extensive damage to your trees and foliage. The now dead or dying trees may attract other insects which will infest the yard and cause even more damage. The once beautiful yard may be forever changed.

This is essentially what happens in our gut whenever we take certain drugs, particularly antibiotics. The antibiotics, like the pesticides, kill bacteria indiscriminately, and even the good bacteria fall prey. Without friendly bacteria to protect us, unfriendly organisms, especially yeasts which are not affected by antibiotics, multiply out of control. Unfriendly bacteria find the new surroundings to their liking and establish residence. They grow and multiply. The entire environment of the digestive tract is altered. These unfriendly residents produce waste products that are toxic. Consequently, digestive health is seriously compromised. The result is numerous health problems including constipation, diarrhea, indigestion, heartburn, ulcers, gas, bloating, irritable bowl syndrome, leaky gut syndrome, diverticulitis, hemorrhoids, cancer, and poor nutrient absorption. The problems aren't restricted to just the digestive tract, but affect the entire body. Poisons produced by these troublemakers are absorbed into the intestinal wall and find their way into the bloodstream where they can wreck havoc on the liver, kidneys, heart, joints, and every other organ and tissue in the body. For this reason, researchers have found associations between digestive health and problems such as arthritis, asthma, acne, eczema, rosacea, chronic fatigue, migraines, and depression, to name a few.

The yeast *Candida albicans* is one of the most troublesome inhabitants of our digestive tract. Everybody hosts candida to one extent or another and ordinarily it poses little threat. In a healthy digestive tract populated with friendly bacteria, candida behaves itself, causing no problems. However, if you remove the good guys by killing them off with medications and poor diet, these once benign yeast cells transform into a hideous fungus that terrorizes the digestive tract. Candida undergoes a Dr. Jekyll and Mr. Hyde type of transformation. As a yeast cell, the Dr. Jekyll form of candida is essentially harmless. But given the opportunity in the right environment it can quickly transform into a multi-celled mycelial form of fungus—the Mr. Hyde form. In this form candida sprouts root-like projects called rhizoids which penetrate into the intestinal wall, creating inflammation and interfering with nutrient absorption.

Like trees growing along a street whose roots fracture and break the concrete sidewalk, the intestinal wall is fractured by rhizoids. Many health care professionals believe this is what causes leaky gut syndrome and many types of food allergies. Incompletely digested food proteins, which are ordinarily too large to pass through the intestinal wall, are now able to enter and eventually find their way into the bloodstream. These "foreign" proteins in the blood are regarded as invaders by the immune system, which mounts a feverish attack to eliminate them. The consequence is allergic symptoms.

Probiotics

Probiotics do many things to protect us from harmful micoflora and keep us healthy. One of their primary duties is to help us digest food and improve nutrient absorption. Much of the plant food we eat contains complex carbohydrates that we cannot digest. We call this *dietary fiber*. We do not produce the enzymes necessary to break these carbohydrates into smaller units. However, intestinal bacteria do. They feed on the fiber and in the process create vitamins and other nutrients essential to our health.

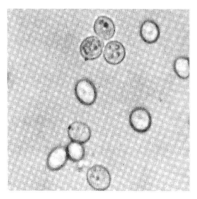

Candida normally live in the digestive tract as individual yeast cells.

Probiotics manufacture a variety of essential nutrients including vitamins B-6, B-12, K, niacin, biotin, folic acid, thiamine (B-1), riboflavin (B-2), and pantothenic acid (B-5). They make important amino acids like arginine, cysteine, and glutamine. They break down complex carbohydrates which we can't ordinarily digest into smaller units that we can then utilize for nourishment.

One of the most important products probiotics manufacture from dietary fiber is short chain fatty acids (SCFA). SCFA are very important to our intestinal health. SCFA are utilized by the cells along the intestinal wall of our digestive tract as food. These small fat molecules are easily absorbed into our cells, providing them with energy. They also perform another very important function—they kill disease causing microorganisms. Just as they are easily absorbed into our intestinal cells, SCFA are also easily absorbed into the cells of certain troublesome bacteria and yeasts, but instead of nourishing them, they cause these organisms to rupture and die. It's sort of like puncturing the skin on a bubble. These organisms simply fall apart. In this way, harmful organisms in our digestive tract are kept under control.

Some friendly bacteria produce antitoxins—substances that inhibit the growth of their less friendly competitors and protect us against the toxins they produce. For instance, *L. acidophilus* produces acidophilin, a substance that is known to have antibiotic effects against at least 22 other strains of bacteria, including *E. coli*, *Shigella dysenteriae*, *Staphylococcus aureus*, *Streptococcus lactis*, and *Salmonella schottmueleri*.

Another way harmful organisms are prevented from proliferating is by the acidic environment within the digestive tract. Friendly bacteria produce lactic acid which lowers pH (acidifies) the gut. Unfriendly organisms find the acidic environment too uncomfortable and, therefore, they tend to keep a low profile. We do the same thing. Human populations are relatively sparse in northern Canada and in the Sahara Dessert. Just as we don't like living in environments that are too cold or too hot, some bacteria and yeasts don't like it too acidic, and few take up residence there.

Probiotics keep our digestive tract healthy and functioning properly. Any disruption in the probiotic population can lower our immunity and reduce our ability to fight off infections. Probiotics block the growth of cancer. Studies show that these microflora help suppress the growth of tumors induced by toxic chemicals. They also inhibit the action of certain enzymes that transform substances into carcinogens. They are especially helpful in protecting against stomach and colon cancer, but have also been shown to protect against breast and other cancers.[1-2]

Probiotics prevent and treat diarrhea and constipation. Much of the research on probiotics has focused on their use as a therapy for diarrheal diseases, especially in children. High colon pH has been linked with constipation, and lowering pH, making it more acid, has been found to relieve this condition.

Probiotics prevent and treat halitosis (bad breath) and body odor. Chronic bad breath and body odor are often the result of an overgrowth of undesirable bacteria in the gastrointestinal tract. These bacteria produce putrefying waste products that circulate throughout the body, producing offensive odors.

Canker sores, stomach ulcers, and some forms of colitis are caused by infections from unfriendly bacteria and viruses. Maintaining the natural balance of the digestive tract keeps these troublemakers at bay. Likewise with inflammatory diseases such as Crohn's disease, ulcerative colitis, and irritable bowel syndrome. All of these conditions are directly related to an imbalance of the body's inner ecosystem.

What Alters Inner Ecology?

Many factors can influence the ecology in our gastrointestinal tract. Diet is one. The over consumption of sugar and processed white flour products promotes the growth of yeasts and bad bacteria. Sugar, in particular, is troublesome because it depresses immune function which is active in suppressing unsavory microflora. The immune system is like our internal police force. They are on constant watch for criminal activity. Wrongdoers are constantly removed from the population. However, when we eat sugar, the police force is, in effect, downsized. With fewer police on duty, more crime is committed. In other words, the bad bacteria are allowed to remain in the population and multiply.

A diet that is low in fresh fruits and vegetables and other healthy foods and heavy in highly processed and packaged foods doesn't supply adequate nourishment to properly feed the body. Consequently, immune function is depressed, which again allows the overgrowth of undesirable microflora.

Anything that depresses immune function can affect our inner ecology, including excessive stress, lack of exercise, lack of sleep, and tobacco and alcohol use. As bad microflora increase, the immune system is put under additional stress, thus compounding the problem.

Drugs and medications affect our inner environment. Antibiotics are the most notorious in this respect, but steroids, estrogens, and even excessive progesterone also have an effect. Antacids cause problems because they reduce acid levels allowing undesirable bacteria, such as *H. pylori,* the bacterium that causes stomach ulcers, to gain a foothold.

THE MAGIC OF CULTURED FOODS

If eating the wrong types of food disrupts the natural ecosystem in our digestive tract, then eating the right kinds of foods will bring it back and help keep it in balance. Fermented foods have long been known for their ability to balance the intestinal environment and promote good health. The reason for this is because they supply a rich source of probiotics.

Fermented or cultured foods have been an important part of the human diet for ages. Sauerkraut, kimchi, kefir, yogurt, and other fermented foods supply a rich source of probiotics. These foods have long been noted for their health promoting properties. They were used to both nourish the body and to prevent and treat illness. Roman armies were kept in the peak of health on a diet of sauerkraut. Dutch seafarers took sauerkraut with them on long ocean voyages to prevent scurvy. The secret to the excellent health and long lifespans of inhabitants of Caucasian mountains of Southern Russia was attributed to kefir—a fermented milk.

Fermented foods, and especially cultured milk, first gained notoriety among the scientific community with the work of Russian scientist Ilya Metchnikoff. Beginning in the 1920s Metchnikoff, a recipient of the Nobel Prize in microbiology, noted the connection between the health of populations and the consumption of yogurt. For instance, Bulgarian peasants whose diet included a great deal of yogurt, were unusually healthy and lived to extraordinary ages. Their good health, claimed

Metchnikoff, came from a diet high in probiotics. He developed the theory that the daily consumption of lactic acid bacteria in cultured milk could fend off disease and prolong life.

Today, fermented foods and probiotic dietary supplements are used to balance the environment in the digestive tract, improve digestive function, and fight candida infections. The health of the colon has a dramatic effect on the health of the entire body. A toxic colon can absorb poisons which are spread throughout the body, causing a variety of reactions not ordinarily associated with the gut, including eczema, migraine headaches, arthritis, cancer, and hormonal imbalances. For this reason, one of the primary goals of natural health practitioners is to balance the digestive tract. Cultured foods are often recommended as part of a healthy diet.

When foods or liquids are allowed to ferment naturally, the culture comes from organisms that happen to be present on the food or in the air. The type of bacteria varies somewhat from place to place and even from season to season. So the organisms in one batch of fermented milk, for example, may differ somewhat from another. The organisms that make kefir, for instance, are different from those in yogurt. Kefir actually contains a mixture of about 50 different bacteria and yeasts. This combination gives kefir its unique flavor. If you wanted to maintain a consistent flavor, you would need to keep a portion of a previous batch to use as the starter culture for the next.

The medium in which the culture grows also affects the type of organisms and the taste of the final product. Milk and fruit juice are the traditional favorites for fermentation. But even plain water can be used if sugar and a culture are added. Coconut water is like a fruit juice and can be used to make a variety of cultured drinks.

Coconut water makes an ideal fermentation medium. It is rich in sugars, which are needed to feed the lactic acid bacteria involved in the fermentation process. In addition to sugar it contains inulin, a dietary fiber made of fructose molecules. Inulin is a favorite food for lactic acid bacteria and stimulates their growth. In fact, it's like a fertilizer for gut bacteria. It is often sold as a dietary supplement under the names inulin, fructooligosaccharide, or FOS. Coconut water also contains plant growth hormones that stimulate bacteria growth. With all this probiotic stimulus, coconut water naturally begins to ferment once it has been exposed to the bacteria in the air. Cultured coconut water is a living water because it is teeming with live beneficial bacteria.

Coconut water can be cultured to produce a variety of products depending on the culture used and the flavoring agents. In the Philippines a favorite type of cultured coconut water is *nata de coco*. Coconut farmers make it at home and combine it with fruit and eat it as a dessert. It has a mild flavor, a translucent gelatin-like appearance, and a chewy texture—kind of like a gummy bear. Unlike cultured dairy, it is a good source of dietary fiber. The fiber is from bacterial cellulose, which gives it its distinctive chewy texture. It is considered a health food in the Philippines because it is a rich source of fiber and low in calories. Since it has nearly zero calories, it makes an ideal bulk diet food. It can help fill you up without filling you out. It is also reported to prevent gastrointestinal disorders and colon cancer, and has even been used as a dressing for wounds. Although it originated in the Philippines, it has become immensely popular in Japan and other Asian countries.

In the following sections you will learn how to make your own cultured coconut water products including coconut kefir, lacto-fermented coconut water ginger ale, and other flavored beverages.

COCONUT WATER KEFIR

Traditionally kefir is made with milk. For those who do not wish to eat dairy or who follow a vegan lifestyle, kefir can be made using fruit juice or coconut water. A culture designed specifically for this purpose is a water kefir called tibicos. You can use traditional kefir or tibicos to make coconut water kefir. Coconut water kefir is a tasty, fizzy, tart, yet mildly sweet beverage.

Donna Gates, author of the *Body Ecology Diet*, recommends coconut water kefir as a means of cleansing the body and helping to restore and maintain the body's inner ecology. She reports that it helps people improve their complexion, stop sugar cravings, ease aches and joint pains, improve vision, balance hormones, increase energy, and produce an overall feeling of good health. The combination of coconut water's natural benefits with those of probiotics makes this a powerhouse health drink.

Kefir cultures are referred to as *grains* because of their grainy appearance. A large culture looks something like a small head of

Sugar Cravings

I have tried unsuccessfully to lose weight for over 10 years. Along came young coconut kefir and I have lost my weight effortlessly. From the first day I started drinking young coconut kefir my sugar cravings left and I haven't eaten any sugar since. I have lost 50 pounds and follow the Body Ecology Diet without problems. I had no idea I would lose as much as I have in a short period of time. Before I began young coconut kefir I was sick all the time. I am healthy now. It is definitely a miracle.

Martha

cauliflower. The texture of the grains is rubbery. Once you purchase some kefir grains you can keep your culture alive indefinitely. As the kefir ferments, the grains grow and multiply. Once the beverage is fermented and ready to consume, the grains are removed and used to make the next batch.

A more convenient and somewhat easier method of making kefir is to use a starter packet. The contents of the packet, which is a powder, is put into the liquid and fermented. Kefir grains do not develop, so you need to reserve some of the liquid from one batch to use as the starter for the next batch. This way there are no grains to worry about or filter out. However, with each new batch of kefir you make, the composition of the microorganisms change slightly. So after you've made 6-7 batches the taste is noticeably different and you have to start over again with a new packet.

Kefir grains or starter packets are available at health food stores or online. Making kefir is easy. Fill a *glass* quart jar with coconut water. Mason jars work perfectly. Pour the kefir starter (grains or packet) into the coconut water. Put a lid on the jar; it doesn't have to be screwed on tight, its purpose is to keep out dust and bugs. Place the jar in a spot away from sunlight, such as a cupboard. Let it ferment for 24-48 hours. The time needed depends on the temperature; the warmer it is, the quicker the fermentation. As it ferments, the water turns a somewhat milky white with a few bubbles forming on the top. When the kefir is ready to drink, it will have a pleasant, tangy taste. The microorganisms in the water feed on the sugar, so the longer it ferments, the more sour it becomes. It can transform from mildly sweet and tangy to sour overnight so don't ignore it. To stop fermentation, put the coconut kefir into the refrigerator. This action will not completely prevent further fermentation but will slow it down considerably. You can store it the refrigerator for several weeks without problem. If you plan on storing it for a long time, you might want to add a tablespoon or so of sugar for the organisms to feed on.

If you use kefir grains, filter out the grains and add them to your next batch. If you use kefir starter, reserve about a half cup (the amount doesn't need to be exact) of the current batch and use it as your starter for the next quart of coconut kefir. The size and number of grains or the amount of starter you use will affect the speed at which the next batch ferments. The more you use, the faster the fermentation.

If the climate you are in is cool, it may take longer to ferment. To speed up the process, warm the liquid to about 90 degrees F (32 C) before adding the kefir starter. Wrap the jar for insulation and place in a warm spot. Fermentation proceeds best at temperatures above 65 degrees F (18 C).

A Natural Chelator

My 7-year-old son has autism, and was diagnosed with heavy metal poisoning and gut dysbiosis. I came across the Body Ecology Diet, and read about young coconut kefir being a natural chelator and helping with digestion. We started to see changes immediately. His distended stomach started to become flat. He began having regular bowel movements that were normal looking. His excessive hunger started to go away. I didn't tell any of his teachers or therapists that he was taking young coconut kefir, but they all started noticing changes too. The dark circles under his eyes started to vanish, he is happier and more focused when doing tasks, and started communicating more with others. He has become a healthier child since taking young coconut kefir. I wish I had known about it sooner.

Jackie

Eczema

My son got his first symptoms of eczema when he was two months old. At 1½ years old, over 90 percent of his body was covered in eczema. My son had the skin of an alligator. We began to notice a cycle of behavior changes, sleeplessness, and eczema flares and this really scared me. Our breaktrhough came after we found a local Asian market that sold young green coconuts. I began to use the Body Ecology Diet kefir starter to kefir the young green coconut water. Now we might go weeks without any eczema flare-ups at all and his skin is as soft as any other young child's. You have no idea what it feels like to hold him in my lap without having to brace myself for the feeling of his skin. He is happy and calm and playful again.

Angie

LACTO-FERMENTED COCONUT WATER

In times past, people preserved foods for long periods without the use of refrigerators or freezers. This was done through the process of lacto-fermentation. Lactic acid is a natural preservative that inhibits the growth of less friendly bacteria and yeasts. Sugars in foods and beverages are converted into lactic acid by lactic-acid-producing bacteria. These bacteria are present everywhere. They are in the soil, on plants, and even in the air. Lacto-fermentation is the process that turns cabbage into sauerkraut and cucumbers into pickles. It can also be used to make lacto-fermented beverages. Sodas such as ginger ale and root beer were originally produced by lacto-fermentation. Coconut water makes an excellent base for making lacto-fermented soda the old fashioned way.

Lacto-fermented coconut water provides many of the same health benefits as coconut water kefir. The primary differences are that the taste is a little different and you don't need to buy a starter, you make your own. Also, you can make a variety of flavors including ginger ale and root beer, an excellent alternative to commercially produced soda high in sugar and loaded with preservatives and who knows what.

Basically all you do is combine coconut water, sugar, and a culture and let it ferment. The following directions produce 1 quart of lacto-fermented coconut water soda. Flavoring can be added, but is optional.

Starter Culture

Begin by making a starter culture. You will need a 1 pint (475 ml) or larger glass jar. A pint size Mason jar is perfect. Fill the jar with 1 pint of filtered or distilled water. Do not use chlorinated tap water. Chlorine kills the bacteria. If you have to use tap water, boil it first for about five minutes or let the water stand for 24 hours to evaporate out the chlorine.

Take a piece of fresh ginger about 1 inch long and cut it into very thin slices. Trim off and discard any mold. Mold will sometimes grow where the ginger has previously been cut or broken. You do not need to peel the skin off the ginger. The skin contains lactic acid bacteria that will help develop your culture. Put the ginger slices into the jar of water. Add 2 teaspoons of white sugar. Cover the jar with a cloth to keep out dust and bugs and put it in a dark location, such as a cupboard. Let the ginger water ferment for about seven days. Stir in 1 teaspoon of sugar every day while it is fermenting. During this time the beverage should become bubbly and have a pleasant odor.

If some funky colored growth develops in the culture, it is mold; scoop it out and continue. You can dump the whole thing out and start again, but you don't need to. I generally just scoop the mold out and keep the rest of the culture. Sometimes mold will grow on the mat of bacteria that often develops on the surface of the liquid. As long as the mold is just on the surface, it's okay. Remove it and continue.

Putting It Together

You have enough starter culture to make 2 or more quarts of soda. Put about ½ cup (120 ml) of the starter culture into a 1 quart (950 ml) glass jar. You can use more or less of the starter culture if you like, but more gives the lactic acid bacteria a head start over other fermentation organisms, such as alcohol-producing yeasts. Add ¼ cup (60 ml) of sugar. The sugar is optional, but it feeds the lactic acid bacteria and encourages their growth and enhances the flavor of the final product. You can use almost any form of sugar—white sugar, brown sugar, sucanat, maple sugar, coconut sugar, or rice syrup. You can also use molasses but I don't recommend it because the flavor is too strong for most people. Honey is not recommended. It possesses antibacterial properties that inhibit fermentation. I prefer to use sucanat (dehydrated sugarcane juice) because it gives the beverage a delicious caramel-like flavor. Sucanat is available at most health food stores. Fill the rest of the jar with coconut water. Put a lid on the jar. The lid can be loose or tight; it works either way. I like to screw the lid on tight because it keeps the carbonation in, giving it more fizz. During fermentation carbon dioxide gas, which makes the soda fizzy, is formed. If you put the lid on tight, pressure will build and it will pop a bit when you release it, just like a bottle of soda. As it ferments, it will turn cloudy and a few bubbles will form on the top. When it does this, you know that the lactic acid bacteria are happy.

Store the jar in a place that is always kept dark. Sunlight tends to kill the microorganisms. Let it ferment for 2-5 days, depending on the temperature. If temperatures in the room reach 70 degrees F (21 C) or more during the day, the beverage may be ready in 2 days. Lactic acid bacteria eat up the sugar so it becomes less sweet and more tart and fizzy with time. You can drink it at any stage.

Once it has reached a point where you want fermentation to stop, either drink it or put it into the refrigerator. Cold dramatically slows down the fermentation process. You can keep it in the refrigerator for several weeks.

Reserve about half a cup of the previous batch to serve as the starter for the next batch. You can continue this process indefinitely. If you aren't going to be making a new batch for some time, you can keep a portion in the refrigerator for many weeks and even months. Add a tablespoon or so of sugar to feed the bacteria. Although fermentation slows down, the bacteria are alive and need nourishment. If you're not going to make the drink again for an extended time, you can just start from the beginning with a new culture.

Flavored Drinks

The basic drink described above is delicious in its own right, but you can create variety by adding different flavorings. The basic lacto-fermented coconut water described has a ginger ale like flavor because of the ginger starter culture. However, as additional batches are made, the ginger taste becomes increasingly diluted so by the second or third batch the ginger flavor is essentially gone. The fermented coconut water tastes good with no added flavors but, if you desire, you can spice it up. The flavorings are the same as our ancestors used—herbs and spices. Besides ginger you can use sarsaparilla, sassafras, licorice root, cinnamon, vanilla bean, nutmeg, anise, coriander, allspice, and mint, to name a few. Medicinal herbs can also be used if you want a particular health benefit associated with a certain herb, but these beverages often have an herbal medicine-like taste. Ginger makes a great ginger ale drink and sarsaparilla and sassafras produce a root beer flavor. Have fun and experiment with different herbs and spices.

If you have an extract such as vanilla or mint, you can simply add that to the product either before or after fermentation. If you don't have an extract, you need to make your own. If you are using delicate herbs, such as flowers or leaves, bring a cup of coconut water or plain water to a boil, remove from heat and seep the herbs in the hot water for about 5 minutes. For root, stem, seed, and bark herbs, bring 1 cup (240 ml) of water to a boil, cover, and simmer the herbs in the water for about 15-20 minutes. Chopping the herbs into small pieces allows more of the flavor to seep into the water. Use the same amount of herbs you would use to make about 4 cups of tea. You will end up with 1 cup of very strong tea. It needs to be stronger than ordinary tea because you are going to dilute it with the other ingredients.

Remove the herbs and let the flavoring cool. Combine ¼ to ½ cup (60-120 ml) of flavoring with culture, coconut water, and sugar into a 1 quart (950 ml) jar and continue with the fermentation procedure previously described.

Overview

The process of making lacto-fermented coconut water can be boiled down into a few simple steps.

Initial Batch

Step 1: Prepare culture starter. Combine chopped or sliced ginger with 1 pint (475 ml) of water and 2 teaspoons (10 ml) sugar. Add 1 teaspoon of sugar every day. Cover and store in a dark spot for 7 days. This makes enough starter for 4 or more quarts.

Health Conditions Influenced by Our Inner Ecology

Acne	Heartburn
Asthma	Headaches/Migraines
Bad Breath	Hemorrhoids
Body Odor	Indigestion
Yeast Infection/Candidiasis	Irritability
Canker Sores	Irritable Bowel Syndrome (IBS)
Colitis	Leaky Gut Syndrome
Constipation	Low Immunity/Frequent
Crohn's Disease	Infections
Depression	Psoriasis
Diarrhea	Rheumatoid Arthritis
Eczema	Rosacea
Fatigue	Skin and Toenail Fungus
Food Allergies	Ulcers
Gas, Flatulence, Bloating	

If you experience any of the above conditions, it is likely that the environment in your digestive tract needs attention. Reestablishing a healthy intestinal ecology may be the key factor in overcoming these problems. Dietary changes, including the addition of coconut water, can help to reestablish a healthy inner ecology.

Step 2: Combine ½ cup (120 ml) of starter culture with ¼ cup (60 ml) sugar, and enough coconut water to fill a 1 quart (950 ml) glass container.

Step 3: Fermentation. Put a lid on the jar and store in a warm, dark spot for 2-5 days.

Step 4: Drink and enjoy. Save some to start the next batch.

Subsequent Batches

Step 1: Use about ½ cup (120 ml) of the previous batch as your starter.

Step 2: Make flavoring (optional). Bring 1 cup (240 ml) of coconut water or plain water to a boil. To extract flavor from flowers and

153

leaves, seep in hot water for 5 minutes. For other herbs, simmer for 15-20 minutes. Let cool before combining with other ingredients.

Step 3: Mix ingredients together. Combine ½ cup of starter culture with ¼ to ½ cup (60-120 ml) flavoring (optional), ¼ cup (60 ml) sugar, and enough coconut water to fill a 1 quart (950 ml) glass container.

Step 4: Fermentation. Put a lid on the jar and store in a warm, dark spot for 2-5 days.

Step 5: Drink and enjoy. Start the next batch.

COCONUT VINEGAR

Coconut vinegar is very popular in the tropics, partly because it is so easy to make. Coconut vinegar can be made from both coconut water or tree sap (toddy). All you need to do is let it ferment. That's it. In the Philippines it is sold everywhere: in stores, by street venders, and on roadside stands in the country. Coconut vinegar, like apple cider vinegar, is legendary for its health benefits and multiple uses. Coconut vinegar has a very delightful taste that can spark up salads, pasta, and other foods.

To make coconut vinegar from coconut water the best way is with a starter culture. You can get the culture from almost any commercial organic apple cider vinegar, such as Spectrum or Braggs. Although these products are bottled, they contain live cultures or will as soon as they are opened and exposed to the air. Use 1 tablespoon of apple cider vinegar for every cup (240 ml) of fresh coconut water. Let the mixture ferment in a dark location for 2-4 weeks until it becomes vinegary. You do not need to add sugar.

The coconut vinegar will grow a culture of bacteria that will float on top of the water. This mat of bacteria is translucent with a soft jelly-like texture. This is called the "mother of vinegar." Remove the mother and use it as the starting culture for the next batch. The mother can be stored in the refrigerator with some coconut water or sugar water to keep it nourished. It will last indefinitely as long as it has a source of nourishment. Homemade vinegar need not be stored in the refrigerator but you can if you want to retard further fermentation.

8

Coconut Water Detox

A NEW LIFE

"I'm dying!" exclaimed 34-year old Jack Goldstein. In spite of his training as a medical doctor, Jack was a sick man.

After six years of suffering, Jack had run the gamut of medical treatment and by all standards there wasn't much hope left for him. He suffered from ulcerative colitis, a severe and debilitating disease of the colon (large intestine) marked by severe diarrhea, intestinal spasms, bleeding, dehydration, weakness, weight loss, and a host of other symptoms. It is one of the chronic digestive diseases which, according the National Center for Health Statistics, are the number one cause of hospitalization and rank second as the cause of disability due to illness.

It was at this point the doctor offered him two choices: 1) do nothing and die, or 2) undergo a drastic operation, a total colectomy (complete removal of the five or six feet of the large intestine and rectum), with a bag being attached to the abdomen for the collection and elimination of waste matter, which would have made him a permanent cripple, and would not guarantee his survival.

Jack's nightmare began six years earlier when he was 28 years old and had been in private practice only three and one-half years. "My wife, Corinne, and I were relaxing one evening after supper, when suddenly and without warning came a feeling of pressure and discomfort in my lower abdomen, accompanied by strong urge to have a bowel movement. It happened so fast, there was no time to reach the lavatory and I found myself sitting in a small pool of blood, the sight of which worried and frightened me."

After the initial shock wore off, he decided to do nothing for the time being. After all, he didn't seem to have any other health problems. Over the next three weeks diarrhea developed, accompanied by bleeding and intestinal spasms. This prompted him to make an appointment to see a specialist. The diagnosis was ulcerative colitis and treatment began. Over the next six years he took some 40 different types of medications, gulping down combinations of half a dozen varieties at a time, which caused reactions that, in Jack's words, "made the ulcerative colitis look like child's play." Diet was also regimented consisting of low-fiber, mostly over-cooked soft foods to prevent irritating his already sensitive intestinal lining.

It wasn't just his digestive tract that was affected, his entire body was sick. What is sometimes overlooked is the fact that the body is one unit. One cannot isolate a part and say this is the sick portion. When one part is diseased or ails in some way, the body as a whole is sick.

There were periodic improvements followed by flare-ups, until eventually there were more flare-ups than improvements and the disease became chronic and crippling. "There were days when I could not go to work. There were days when I was in my office and did not have the strength to stay more than few hours before I found it necessary to go home and drop into bed. There were also days where I awoke in the morning and could not get out of bed."

Diarrhea gradually increased to about 30 times a day, much of it just intestinal spasms and bleeding. His rectal area became extremely sore and painful hemorrhoids developed due to the constant spasms from the diarrhea. The inability to properly digest and absorb nutrients from foods contributed to malnourishment. He lost 30 pounds, dropping from 170 to 140. Pains developed that migrated from joint to joint. He was hospitalized several times to combat rampant internal infections and at one point required surgery to remove gangrenous hemorrhoids that were literally rotting away on his body.

It became increasingly difficult for him to maintain his medical practice and to have a social life. "My life now was completely revolving around my problems almost to the exclusion of anything else," Laments jack. "Whenever my wife and I would go anywhere, my first objective was to locate the lavatory and stay within close range. I was living in constant fear and under heavy stress because of never knowing when or where or how fast the urge would strike. I didn't live from week to week, day to day, hour to hour or even minute to minute. I lived from second to second."

He went to specialist after specialist to find a solution, without luck. Deep depression set in. The future looked bleak. "I could only foresee a futile struggle to exist…my physical and psychological debility worsening until I became a complete invalid (if I lived that long)."

Finally his doctor told him that there was nothing more they could do. The only thing left was to surgically remove the entire large intestine and rectum. "I needed time to think. He told me not to wait too long." The thought of radical surgery and being sentenced to a life attached to a waste collection bag was frightening.

"I continued to receive various suggestions from well-meaning people: 'Go to the Mayo Clinic,' or 'Go to the Cleveland Clinic,' or 'I know a famous doctor in New York.' Frankly, I didn't want any more advice. I was tired of it. I had run the medical gamut and just did not have the desire, stamina, or money to run it again. I also did not want to submit to some of the 'heroic' methods being used. I don't believe I could have survived it."

Jack's wife suggested he look into alternative therapies and told him about a local vegetarian organization which had a small library on alternative health and diet. Jack refused. "As far as I was concerned, this was some sort of quackery, chicanery. I would not even open my mind enough to read any literature on the subject. After all, I thought, I'm a doctor. What could possible be in those books I don't already know?"

Over the next several weeks his wife persisted in asking him to check it out. Jack continued to resist. His doctor kept pushing for the surgery. Perhaps out of desperation more than anything else, Jack finally summoned the courage to check out the books. He came away with four books by Dr. H. M. Shelton, one of which was titled *Fasting Can Save Your Life*. "I immediately opened and began reading, defensively I might add. But soon this defensiveness disappeared and the gates of my mind swung open. This book was not only fascinating, it was thought provoking, enlightening, and it made sense. For the first time in six years I was truly motivated. I couldn't put the book down."

He made up his mind to try the methods described in the book. There was nothing to lose and everything to gain. He reasoned that if the treatment failed he could still have the operation. Delaying the operation a few more months wouldn't make much difference. So he contacted a health clinic in New York which had experience in fasting therapy and dietary modification.

He was assigned a room at the clinic and immediately put on a fast for the next six weeks, consuming nothing but water. All drugs were discontinued. Although emaciated from his six year struggle, the lack of nutrition on his fast did not adversely affect him.

Over the next 42 days he went through the process of detoxification with various episodes of discomfort as toxins were expelled through his bowels, mouth, nose, and skin. In the beginning he experienced low back pain, dehydration, foul breath, insomnia, and, of course, hunger with thoughts of food constantly in his mind. Although abstaining from all food, and taking only water, bowel activity continued, gradually diminishing until the last few days of the fast. As periods of cleansing came and went he began to feel better and experience a new surge of energy.

At one point a thick foul mucous drained from his sinuses all day, afterwards resulting in the clearest breathing he had in years. He could taste remnants of drugs he had been taking for the past six years as they were expelled from his body. His skin took on a healthy tone and texture. Multiple small warts and other skin blemishes completely disappeared. Tartar and plaque were gone from his teeth, and his gums were now a healthy pink and no longer bleed after vigorous brushing. Best of all, his hemorrhoids were gone, as well as his diarrhea and intestinal pain. Despite losing an additional 32 pounds during the fast, he felt fantastic both physically and mentally, exclaiming "For the first time in years I feel alive!"

Gradually breaking his fast eating mostly fruits and vegetables, he experienced his first normal (non-runny) bowel movement in six years. He began eating whole grains, salads, and raw fruits and vegetables—high fiber foods he was told he would never eat again. He felt as if he had a rebirth. This experience made such an impact on Jack's life he wrote a book about it and became a leading advocate for fasting therapy.[1]

FASTING THERAPY

Fasting is the single most effective form of detoxification. It is nature's way of revitalizing and healing the body. Animals instinctively fast when ill. We too often lose the desire to eat when we are not feeling well. This is the body's way of telling us that it prefers not to be burdened with processing foods as it is battling an infection or some other crisis. The body wants to channel all of its energy into healing.

The body is a marvelous organism. It has the innate ability to recover and heal from just about any affliction. It can do so if not loaded with poisons or torn down by abuse. A doctor may prescribe medication to combat an infection, but he cannot kill the invading microbe. He may suture and bandage an injury, but he cannot heal the wound. He may bring the ends of broken bones together and set them, but he cannot fuse the two sections permanently together. The killing of the virus, healing of the wound, and knitting of the bone along with thousands of other processes involved in the maintenance of our health are things only the body can accomplish. Man cannot duplicate or even imitate the body's remarkable power to heal—he can only assist in the process.

We are subjected daily to a multitude of harmful elements in the foods we eat, the fluids we drink, the air we breathe, and the chemicals we put on our skin, hair, and mouths. Poisons are also generated inside our bodies; some come from the normal processes of metabolism while others come from microorganisms. Poor diet and excessive stress weaken the body and make it more susceptible to health destroying influences.

These negative influences often overwhelm us to the point that disease results. Removing these influences restores health. Fasting can do that. Fasting is not a cure, it is a means by which we assist the body in ridding itself of accumulated filth and allow it to focus its energies on healing and rebalancing.

By definition, fasting is the complete voluntary avoidance of all food and drink. The strictest form of therapeutic fasting allows only the consumption of water. More liberally, it includes fruit and vegetable juices and herbal teas.

Fasting is the oldest therapeutic treatment known to man. It is described in medical texts from ancient Egypt and Greece. Hippocrates, the father of medicine, was a proponent of fasting as a means of restoring good health. In almost every culture, fasting has been used to improve mental, spiritual, or physical well-being.

Fasting therapy has become popular among alternative medical practitioners because of its long history of success and its complete independence from drugs and invasive therapies. It is currently used extensively in Europe and Asia and to a lesser degree in the United States. Published medical studies and clinical observation have found fasting to be effective in treating a number of health problems including some hard to treat conditions such as ulcerative colitis and cancer. Some of the conditions that respond well to fasting therapy include arthritis, eczema, psoriasis, cysts, migraines, tinnitus, irritable bowel syndrome, varicose veins, gallbladder disease, hypertension, fibromyalgia, obesity, chronic back pain, allergies, autoimmune disorders, and cardiovascular diseases.[2-6]

While it has proven useful, it does have some drawbacks. The biggest hurdle to fasting is the discomfort associated with going without food for an extended period of time. Physically and psychologically it is very difficult. Most people don't have the determination or willpower to undergo an extended fast, particularly a water fast. It usually takes a health crisis like a serious chronic illness or the threat of radical surgery to motivate someone to keep with it for any length of time.

During a *water* fast, a number of undesirable side effects often occur. One of which is dehydration. Although water consumption is encouraged, the desire to drink greatly diminishes. Water is lost from urine, bowels, skin, and respiration—about 108 ounces (3200 ml) a day, even when fasting. Adequate hydration is very important during detoxification. Water acts as the medium in which toxins are dissolved and flushed out of the body. If the body is dehydrated it will want to hold onto the water to prevent further dehydration, thus limiting the amount of toxins expelled.

Accompanying dehydration is an electrolyte imbalance. As fluids are removed from the body, electrolytes are taken with them. If pure water is the only fluid consumed electrolyte deficiencies will develop. The first sign of depleted electrolytes is a loss of the desire to drink. Water no longer quenches thirst and takes on a mildly unpleasant taste. This is the body trying to discourage water consumption because drinking water will further dilute the electrolyte concentration in the body. Since water becomes less appealing, not enough is consumed to replenish what is lost, thus enhancing the effects of dehydration. As the situation worsens it may cause vomiting and dry heaves or expelling bile. This is often experienced in long water fasts.

Constipation also occurs. The combination of dehydration and no food essentially puts the brakes on bowel elimination. However, the bowels may still contain undigested food, mucus, bacteria, and rotten fecal material. Since nothing is eaten to push out this material, it sits. The bowels are a major organ of elimination. When constipated, toxins are stuck and often reabsorbed into the body. For this reason, many fasting advocates recommend daily enemas during the fasting period to emulsify and remove this material.

Since no form of nourishment is consumed there is the potential for developing nutrient deficiencies, especially in extended fasts. While clear signs of nutrient deficiencies such a scurvy, pellagra, and beriberi rarely occur, even during long fasts, nutrient reserves shrink. Minerals which make up the major electrolytes are definitely depleted as well as important vitamins and antioxidants.

The lack of nutrition during water fasts actually slows down the body's ability to heal. Wounds on the surface of the skin, for example, take two or three times as long to heal during a water fast as they normally would.

The absence of consuming energy-producing nutrients (carbohydrate, protein, fat) forces the body to use stored energy reserves. Most of the energy needs are supplied by burning body fat. Consequently, fasting can result in the reduction in body weight of about 1-2 pounds (0.5-1 kg) a day. For most people this is a good thing; the down side is that metabolism slows down and body temperature drops, causing cold hands and feet and a general overall lack of warmth. If the weather is cool the cold is intensified. The drop in metabolism and lack of energy creates a feeling of lethargy. Ordinary tasks become taxing and the slightest physical exertion causes exhaustion. Much of the time is spent resting and napping. When bedtime comes, excessive rest makes nighttime sleep brief and intermittent.

The lack of physical activity causes muscles to atrophy. Lean tissues are cannibalized to help supply the body's need for energy. Muscle mass is reduced.

Despite all these drawbacks, fasting therapy has proven to be a useful tool in restoring health and balancing the body.

Because of the drawbacks mentioned above, water fasts have given way to juice fasting. Fresh fruit and vegetable juices supply an ample source of nutrition without the calories. As a consequence, the body can avoid dehydration, electrolyte and nutrient depletion, and maintain a higher level of energy. Detoxification works faster and more efficiently, with less discomfort.

You will get hunger pangs at first, your energy level will decrease somewhat, you will lose weight, toxins will be purged, but cellular growth and rejuvenation will continue. Juice supplies the body with the needed nutrients to repair damaged tissue and regain health in a shorter amount of time.

COCONUT WATER FAST

Fruit and vegetable juices have been used very successfully in detoxification and fasting therapy. However, one major drawback to juice fasting is the relatively high sugar content of the beverages often used. Sugar feeds undesirable organisms in the intestinal tract, such as candida, and depresses immune function. When people juice fast they generally rely heavily on fruit or carrot juice, both of which are high in sugar. Juices made with only vegetables are overpowering and not particularly pleasant. Have you tried drinking a glass of cabbage juice? Even mild vegetables such as celery can take on an overwhelmingly strong flavor when juiced. Combining the different juices doesn't help. For this reason, fruit or carrot juice is added to tone down the flavor of vegetable juices and make them more palatable. Tomato based juices such as V-8 juice, which can be very appetizing, may contain less sugar, but some people try to avoid nightshade family produce (tomatoes, peppers, eggplant) because they can cause sensitivities and allergic-like reactions.

People who drink a lot of sweet juices, whether fasting or not, may gain some benefit, but end up with a candida infection or have trouble with blood sugar control. To avoid these problems juice fasting utilizes diluted juices along with ample amounts of water. This way both the sugar and calorie content is kept relatively low. Unfortunately,

SUGAR CONTENT IN JUICES		
Juice (1 cup)	Sugar (g)	Calories (kcal)
Coconut Water	6.26	46
Vegetable Cocktail	7.99	46
Tomato	8.65	41
Carrot	9.23	94
Grapefruit	22.48	96
Orange	20.83	112
Apple	27.03	117
Pineapple	31.43	130
Grape	35.27	142

Source: USDA National Nutrient Database for Standard Reference (2006).

when the juices are diluted, the vitamin and mineral content is reduced as well.

As a fasting advocate, I've experimented with juicing many different types of vegetables to produce a juice that is tasty, yet low in sugar and high in nutrition. Without using fruit, carrots, or tomatoes, I have had no success. I began to believe it to be impossible. Until, that is, I discovered coconut water. Coconut water provides the perfect answer. It is lower in sugar and total calories than most fruit, as well as many vegetable juices, supplies a mix of nutrients, and tastes good!

I am no stranger to fasting. I have participated in many water and juice fasts ranging from 1 to 30 days in duration. I have found coconut water to be superior to both water and juice fasting. Coconut water provides all the advantages that juice fasting has over water fasting with many significant additional benefits.

One of the biggest advantages of coconut water is the level of energy it gives as compared to water and juice fasting. During a water fast energy levels are quite low and any exertion can be physically draining. Juice fasting supplies some energy but you still become tired more quickly than you do when not fasting. Not so with coconut water. Although coconut water contains no more calories than juice, normal energy levels are maintained. You can do just about everything on a coconut fast as you normally do. In fact, from my experience I seem to have more energy even though my calorie consumption, from coconut water, may be less than 300 a day. (Coconut water contains about 5.75 calories per ounce.)

You can go to work, do house and yard work, study, and play just as you normally would without anyone ever knowing you are fasting. You can even continue with an exercise program. In fact, I encourage it. Exercise enhances detoxification, healing, and feelings of well-being. My personal exercise program includes jogging for 25-30 minutes and resistance training with hand weights, sit-ups, push-ups, etc. On weekends I often spend several hours working in the yard. During a coconut water fast I can continue with my daily activities, my exercise program, and yard work without problem. Another advantage of exercise is that because you are actively using your muscles you do not lose any lean muscle mass.

Since you can participate in all of your normal daily activities, rather than sitting or napping during the day, at night when you go to bed you sleep soundly. When you awake, you have energy, your mind is clear, and you are ready to start the new day.

Metabolism usually drops during fasting. However, with coconut water, metabolism seems to remain close to normal. You do not get cold hands or feel chilled like you do with a water or juice fast.

Constipation, which is common during a fast, is less of a problem with coconut water. The water helps move debris along and out of the digestive tract. The fact that coconut water tastes better than water and many juices helps prevent dehydration, which also contributes to constipation.

Another big advantage of using coconut water is all the potassium and other ionic minerals it provides, thus helping to maintain electrolyte balance. This is a major drawback with water fasting and one of the reasons why juices have proven to be superior to water.

HOW TO DO A COCONUT WATER FAST

As expected, fasting involves some degree of discomfort. The stomach groans and growls and may even hurt a bit. This will go away. The first day is the hardest. With each succeeding day hunger diminishes.

After the third day hunger is essentially gone. However, thoughts of food will still enter your mind and tempt you. Keep them out as much as possible. If your stomach rumbles or you are tempted to eat, drink some water instead. This will help to satisfy those urges.

No food, whatsoever, is eaten when fasting. Water, however, is absolutely necessary. The water you use should be filtered or bottled, not tap water. Filtered water is recommended because it is free from chlorine, fluoride, and other chemicals typically added to tap water. When you are doing a fast you don't want to be adding more toxins into your body.

Obviously, if you are doing a coconut water fast you will also include coconut water. I recommend that, if possible, you use water from fresh young coconuts (see next chapter for more information about coconuts). If you can't get fresh young coconuts you can use commercially packaged coconut water. In order to get the benefit from the nutrients in coconut water you need to drink the water from more than just one or two coconuts. I would suggest drinking the liquid from 4 to 8 coconuts a day. This amounts to about 45 to 65 ounces (1320 to 1980 ml) per day. To put this in perspective, 1 cup holds 8 ounces (240 ml). So you would shoot for 5 ½ to 8 cups a day. Four cups equals one quart.

You recall from Chapter 3 that a person loses 13.5 cups (3200 ml) of water a day at normal room temperatures. You are still going to be losing water each day. You need to replenish it. Use a combination of coconut water and plain water to get your daily quota. For example, if you drink 6 cups of coconut water, include 7.5 cups of plain water.

The quantities mentioned above are guidelines and not strict rules you must obey. Drink the amount of fluids with which you feel comfortable. Above all, drink enough to avoid dehydration and to maintain electrolyte levels. It is very easy to become dehydrated when fasting. You can tell if you are dehydrated because your mouth becomes dry and your saliva becomes thick. Also, look at your urine. If it is a dark yellow, you are dehydrated. When properly hydrated it should be a very pale yellow, almost clear.

It is also important to consume an adequate amount of salt each day, especially on a coconut water fast to balance out the potassium in the water. Remember, just like an athlete, as you lose water you also lose sodium, chloride, potassium, and other electrolytes. Most of the electrolytes you need are adequately supplied in the coconut water, but you need additional sodium and chloride. You should consume about ¼ to ½ teaspoon of sea salt each day. Sea salt is recommended because it contains important trace minerals that may be leached out of the body during the fast and it doesn't have any additives that are usually included with ordinary table salt. I don't recommend putting it in your water because it makes the water taste too salty and may make it unpalatable. Simply put a tiny amount on your tongue several times a day and let it dissolve. This is actually very pleasant, especially if you haven't been eating, as it provides some degree of oral satisfaction.

You can tell if you have an electrolyte deficiency if your lower back begins to ache. The pain isn't from your spine but from your kidneys. Another sign is when water no longer quenches your thirst and you lose the desire to drink. During a fast your body is trying to eliminate toxins as efficiently as possible and an adequate amount of water is absolutely necessary for this process. Your natural response should be to have an increased thirst. If you lose your desire to drink or the water becomes unpalatable, your body is trying to prevent further leaching of minerals by suppressing your desire to drink mineral deficient fluids.

All medications should be discontinued. They only cause the body to spend energy working to remove them rather than cleaning house. If you must have a prescription drug, check with your doctor before starting a fasting program.

A tendency some might have when fasting is to want to refrain from all physical activity and sleep much of the time. Physical activity is necessary to keep muscles in shape and body fluids circulating. Blood and lymph must circulate in order to purge toxins from the tissues and remove them for the body. Cleansing will actually be quicker if you keep physically active. This does not mean running a marathon, but moderate exercise like walking or aerobics is highly recommended.

Some people feel, since they are not eating, they will have no energy. So they walk around like zombies and complain that they don't have the strength to do anything. This is more psychological than physical. You can continue to go to work and participate in your normal daily activities.

A big factor in the success of your fast is the attitude of the people you are around, especially your family. Most people are ignorant about the process and benefits of fasting. To them, missing a single meal is the onset of starvation. It is wise not to tell anyone you are on a fast. Most people do not understand fasting and will only give you negative comments. Some will argue with or tease and tempt you. To avoid such problems, simply don't tell anyone.

Almost anyone can fast. Overweight people, since they have more stored fat, can fast a longer time than skinnier people. Even thin people carry a reserve of nutrients in their tissues. They too, can benefit from a fast. For some conditions, however, fasting is not recommended. Obviously those suffering from anorexia or malnutrition should not fast. A pregnant or nursing mother should not fast as she needs nourishment for herself and her baby. If you have a serious health condition, you should first check with your health care provider before attempting a fast.

Therapeutic fasts can last up to 40 days or more. Some have extended for over 100 days. Any extended fast like this should be supervised by a health care professional who is experienced in conducting fasts. If you are doing this on your own, you should limit your first fast to 1-3 days.

Before you start, you first need to determine how long you are going to fast. Then you need to obtain all the coconut water you anticipate using during this time. Buy a little extra in case you end up consuming more than you expected or if you decide to extend your fast. You don't want to start a fast thinking you can buy more as you need it because the store may run out of coconut water while you are in the middle of your fast.

Start off with a one day (24 hours) fast. It can last from dinner one day to dinner the next, or breakfast one day to breakfast the next. For example, if you were going to start your fast Friday night, you would eat dinner and then nothing else for the rest of the night. Don't eat a big dinner to tide you over during the fast. Remember, it is the absence of food that brings about cleansing. Saturday morning continue to fast. Skip breakfast and lunch. You will break your fast by eating dinner Saturday evening. Try to make it a full 24 hours. If you want to extend the fast to 36 hours, skip dinner and break the fast when you eat breakfast on Sunday morning. If you feel up to it you can continue the fast.

Fasting is not a one-time thing you do to gain instant health. And you do not need to jump into a 30-day fast to purge all your toxins at one time. Most people have so many toxins in their bodies that they couldn't endure an extended fast without medical supervision. Fasting should be broken into smaller periods of time and repeated frequently. Then, as the body becomes cleaner, longer fast can be attempted.

It Worked for Me

I tried the coconut detox. I had no serious health problems, but I did have several annoying issues such as chronic psoriasis, back and neck pain, jock itch, and was a bit overweight, nothing major, but issues that I would like resolved. The coconut water detox sounded like a possible solution to some of these problems.

I did the coconut water fast for seven days. I consumed an average of 120 ounces (3549 ml) of fluids a day—56 ounces (1556 ml) of coconut water and 64 ounces (1893 ml) of filtered water. The amount of sea salt I ate varied from day to day but averaged a little over $1/8$ teaspoon. I had bowel movements six out of the seven days, although the last few were very small, which is to be expected since I wasn't eating anything.

During the fast I had much more energy and felt warmer than I had when juice fasting. My mind was very clear and alert, more so than normal. It felt good. By the end of the fast I had lost 7 pounds. My back and neck pain, which I had for several months, was gone. Even my eyesight seemed to improve. The biggest change, however, was with my skin. It became very noticeably smoother and softer; it almost seemed to tingle with renewed health and vitality, perhaps due to improved circulation. My chronic psoriasis cleared up remarkably well over this short amount of time. I would say it was about 90 percent better. Jock itch which had been troubling me for the past few weeks was also gone. I was very pleasantly surprised by the results. I have done juice fasting before and never got as good a result on my skin as I did with coconut water.

Paul

After experiencing a few short 1-3 day fasts you can try doing longer 7-14 day fasts if you like. The more often you fast, the longer you will be able to fast. Also, fasting becomes easier with experience. The body becomes more accustomed to periods of calorie deprivation. Psychologically you are more familiar with the process and it is not such an ordeal. Attitude has a great deal to do with the success of fasting. Don't get into the mind frame that you are depriving yourself and don't tempt yourself by dreaming of roast beef sandwiches and fried potatoes. Make up your mind to stick to the fast. Think positively! Focus your thoughts on the cleansing your body is dong and on the health you are achieving. Avoid all temptations. Avoid going into stores where there is the aroma of enticing foods. Remove yourself from all temptation.

Although you can limit your fast to drinking only coconut water, you certainly don't need to. You can add other juices if you like and even combine coconut water with fruit and vegetable juices to add a variety of nutrients in to your program. An excellent beverage to supplement your fasting is coconut herbal tea (see Chapter 10 for coconut water recipes).

WHAT TO EXPECT

People often complain that fasting doesn't work for them because every time they try it, they get sick, or get a headache, or experience other uncomfortable symptoms. The fact that a person is experiencing these symptoms is a sign that the fast is working and the body is cleansing itself. That's the purpose of fasting—purging the body of filth. Removing this sludge will involve an increase in activity of the organs of elimination—lungs, kidneys, bowels, skin. Fasting is a means of detoxification—accelerated detoxification. You should expect some discomfort. You may experience nausea, headaches, diarrhea, skin rashes, coughing, etc. These are the processes of cleansing. This is often referred to as a *healing crisis*. Let the body complete its job. Be prepared for it. Welcome it. It is a sign of healing and improving health. Once the body has eliminated the toxins you will feel much better, better than you did before the crisis.

Your tongue can reveal how much toxic material is stored in your cells and vital organs. The tongue is a mirror of the membrane system of your body. While fasting, the tongue will become heavily coated, and your breath will take on a strong offensive odor. You can watch the progress of your internal cleansing by observing the coating on your tongue. As it builds up, the body is removing more and more and your breath gets worse. You are likely to also have a strong body odor as toxins are released through your skin and sweat glands. Daily baths will relieve much of this. Do not use deodorants, mouthwash, or perfumes. Wash with mild soap and water. Brush your teeth. If you have to do something about bad breath, rinse your mouth with a three percent solution of hydrogen peroxide.

You may encounter mucus congestion, runny nose, coughing, slight fever, aches, and discharges from your eyes and ears. At first, you might think you are coming down with a cold or flu. You're not; this is part of the cleansing experience.

You may or may not have a full-blown healing crisis during a fast. This will depend on your health and the length of your fast. Whether you have a healing crisis or not, you are still cleansing toxins out of your body. If you experience a healing crisis, you can continue to fast; often that may be the only thing you can do as you might be nauseous. But if the symptoms become too unbearable, the fast may be broken and symptoms will subside as the body channels cleansing energy towards digestion and detoxification decelerates.

When you break your fast you should eat fresh, wholesome foods like fresh fruit and vegetables and whole grain products. Continue to drink plenty of liquids. Avoid highly processed, sugary, and fatty foods as they may make you sick. Eat sensibly. You need to give your digestive tract time to adjust to eating again so don't overload it.

Once you've cleansed your body, now is a good time to focus on eating sensibly and continue your progress. Don't load up on junk foods or you will undo everything you've worked for. One of the common complaints with arthritis sufferers is that the fast will relieve their symptoms but after resuming their regular diet the pain eventually returns. The reason it returns is because they continue to eat the foods that caused the problem in the first place. If after the fast they make better dietary choices and eat healthfully, arthritic symptoms do not come back.[7]

170

9

A Lovely Bunch of Coconuts

THE KING OF JUICES

When I tasted coconut water for the first time, I didn't know what to think. It wasn't at all like I expected. It was slightly sweet with a mild somewhat nutty flavor and didn't taste anything like the shredded coconut with which I was familiar. It was in stark contrast to the highly flavored and sugary fruit juices and sodas we are accustomed to. I liked it. It was refreshing and definitely a healthier choice over commercial beverages.

Since that time I have had coconut water from all over the world. I have found that the taste of the water varies somewhat from place to place due to the different varieties of coconut and also because of the soil and growing conditions. Younger coconuts are tastier than older ones. The best tasting water comes from coconuts that are 7-9 months old. Water from a freshly picked coconut is better than one that was harvested weeks earlier.

Coconut water is one beverage I don't mind giving to the kids because I know it is good for them, and definitely better than soda or powdered mixes. Most juices contain too much sugar and some contain only small amounts or real juice, being flavored by artificial ingredients and the mysterious "natural" flavors that comes from who knows where.

In terms of health benefits, coconut water is the king of juices. Coconut water is unique. There is no other juice like it. It is the only juice that is the liquid endosperm of a plant. Endosperm, as you recall, is the nutrition storehouse which the seed embryo uses to nourish itself at the time of germination. It is packed with a variety of vitamins, minerals, antioxidants, and anti-aging growth factors. While many fresh juices have vitamins and minerals, they don't have the growth factors. Juice from whole coconuts is also a living food. It is completely compatible with the human body and, unlike other fruit or vegetable juices, can be delivered directly into the bloodstream without any adverse reactions. In comparison with all other juices and beverages, it comes out on top. In terms of health benefits, it is truly the king of juices.

WHERE TO FIND YOUNG COCONUT WATER

If you are fortunate enough to live in the tropics, you have ready access to fresh coconuts and young coconut water. Street venders and restaurants often sell young green coconuts with just the top portion chopped off. The water is then sipped out through a straw. After drinking the liquid, the jelly-like meat can be scooped out and eaten with a spoon.

If you are the adventurous type, you can climb a tree and pick your own coconut, assuming you can actually shimmy up the narrow trunk; it is harder than it looks! Once you get to the top of the tree, you may have your choice of 80 or more coconuts of various ages to choose from. How do you tell which are 7-9 months of age? Coconut palms produce fruit bearing stems about once a month. Each stem may contain 5-12 coconuts. The age of each group of coconuts can be determined by counting each stem starting from the youngest (smallest). Full size is reached at about 6-7 months of age. The older coconuts begin to turn brown as they ripen.

If you don't live in the tropics, you can still enjoy the taste and health benefits of coconut water. Nowadays, coconuts and coconut water are shipped all over the world. Even if you live in Fairbanks, Alaska or Medicine Hat, Canada you can enjoy the benefits of young coconut water. The best place to look for fresh young coconut water is at your local health food store. Some restaurants also carry it, particularly those that specialize in natural, organic, or vegetarian cuisine.

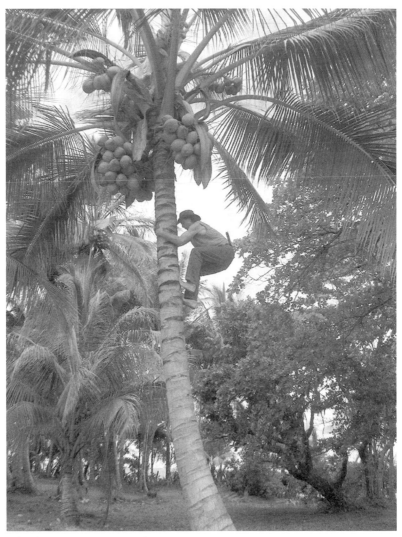

Climbing a coconut palm.

You can find mature coconuts in just about any grocery store. These are the brown hairy ones with which we are most familiar. I don't particularly recommend the water found in these coconuts because they are often cracked and moldy. Besides, even if you do find an

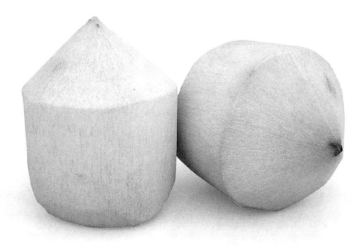

Shaved young coconuts look like large toy tops.

undamaged, uncontaminated mature coconut, the water doesn't compare to that of a young coconut.

Many health food stores, and some groceries, Asian stores, and gourmet shops will carry young coconuts. These coconuts are usually partially dehusked. A coconut with its husk on can be very large, nearly the size of a soccer ball. Cutting off a little excess husk saves space, protects the shell from damage, and allows easier access to the water. These young coconuts are cut into a shape resembling a large toy top. The green skin and much of the inner white husk surrounding the shell is removed. If you have never seen a shaved coconut before, you would wonder what these unusually shaped objects are. They must be kept cool. So you will find them on ice or in a refrigerated compartment at the store.

The shell of young coconuts is thinner and softer than mature coconuts. You can pierce or cut the young shell relatively easily with a knife to access the liquid. One innovative tool on the market to access fresh coconut water is the CocoTap. This little instrument consists of a steel tube with a sharp point at one end and a handle at the other. You simply push the sharp end into the young coconut. It penetrates through

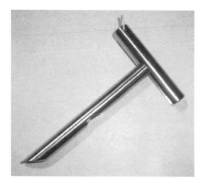

The CocoTap.

the husk and shell. If needed, you can tap the end with a hammer to force it through the shell. The CocoTap is removed from the coconut, leaving a hole. A straw can be inserted into the hole or the liquid can be poured into a glass. It's that simple. The CocoTap works with any unripened coconut. No dehusking is necessary.

Another option available to those who don't live in the tropics is coconut water packaged in a bottle, can, or tetra pak container. The advantage of this type of packaging is long storage life and convenience. You can take it anywhere with you, to the beach, hiking, the gym, or work. Packaged young coconut water is available at most good health food stores and as its popularity increases, it is becoming more widely available in grocery stores.

Once exposed to air, coconut water begins to ferment. In the past, to eliminate microbial growth, commercial bottlers have used high

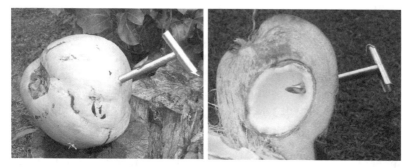

The CocoTap is inserted into a young coconut to access the water. CocoTaps are available online at www.cocotap.com.

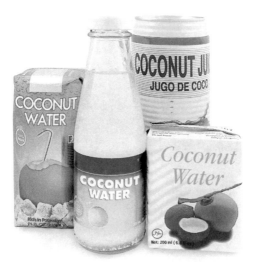

Coconut water is available in convenient, easy-to-carry containers.

temperature, short time pasteurization. In recent years the Food and Agriculture Organization of the United Nations (FAO) has developed a cold sterilization process for coconut water. This process involves no heat so the coconut water remains fresh and vital. The first step in the cold sterilization process is to harvest fresh, unmarred coconuts. Special care is taken to use only freshly harvested coconuts. Coconuts are cut from the trees and lowered to the ground with a rope, not cut and dropped, to avoid the risk of cracking the internal shell. Water collected from coconuts that have dropped to the ground experience a high level of spoilage. The water from bruised coconuts can be consumed within a few hours without problem, but the damage allows microbial growth that will affect the cold sterilization processing, so they are never used in this process. The water in the unopened coconuts is completely sterile and doesn't need any further sterilization. As long as it is not contaminated, it will remain that way. All processing equipment is completely sterilized before it comes into contact with the water. The water is extracted from the coconuts within 24 hours of harvest and immediately refrigerated. It is then filtered to remove solids and particulates, filtered again to remove polyphenols and tannins, and finally sealed in pre-sterilized airtight containers. The final product retains its fresh, natural flavor for 10-12 months. In order to make the cold sterilization process available to as many as possible, the FAO has freely shared this method of production with food processors. It has become one of the most popular methods of packaging coconut water.

HOW TO OPEN A YOUNG COCONUT

The CocoTap is the easiest way by far to access the juice from a young coconut. If you don't have a CocoTap, you can access the water the old fashioned way with a machete! Watch out for your fingers. You have to hit the coconut hard enough to cut through the husk. In the islands, they can do it in three or four quick strikes. A meat cleaver will work as well.

Unless you live in the tropics, the white shaved young coconuts are the type you are most likely to find in the store. They will be on ice or in the refrigerated section. Look for ones that are undamaged and not leaking. A few brown spots are okay. Pick up the coconut and shake it. It should be heavy and you should *not* be able to hear any swishing sound from inside. Young coconuts are completely filled with water. As the coconut matures an air pocket forms as the water is transformed into the meat. When you shake a *mature* coconut, you will hear the water swish around inside. But if you hear that swishing in a young coconut, it is either too old or it is cracked and leaking.

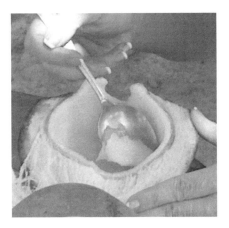

The meat inside young co-conuts is tender and tasty.

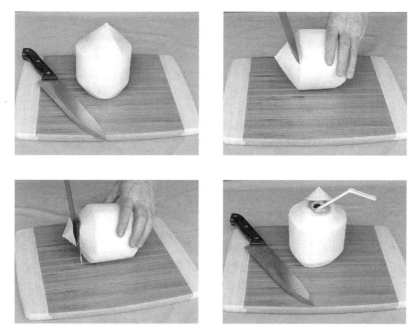

Lay the coconut on its side as shown. With a sharp knife, cut through the end of the coconut using a sawing motion. Cut far enough down from the point to cut into the white meat inside the shell. If the cut is close to the end of the coconut, you will slice through the shell without spilling any of the liquid. You may have to puncture a hole into the meat to access the liquid. Insert a straw and enjoy your drink.

Fortunately, the soft layer of husk surrounding the young coconut does a good job of protecting it from damage.

After you bring your young shaved coconuts home, store them in the refrigerator. Most of these coconuts come from overseas so when you get them, they are already several weeks old. A young coconut will keep for well over a month, if refrigerated. So when you get one at the store, you can keep it for another week or so, but the sooner you consume it the better.

Don't just drink the water and throw the rest away, eat the soft meat as well. The meat gets harder as the coconut matures so you

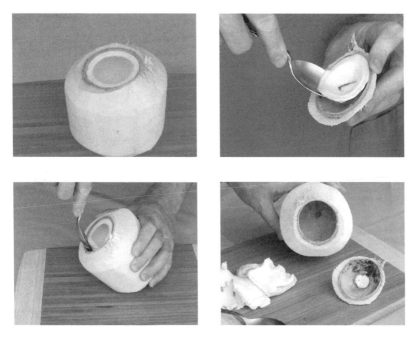

After drinking the liquid, you can remove and eat the soft coconut meat inside the shell. The opening in the coconut needs to be large enough to spoon out the meat. If the hole is too small, cut a larger opening. The meat comes off the shell easily.

may notice some variation in hardness of the meat from one coconut to the next. Very young coconuts 7-8 months old have very soft meat. Coconuts 9-10 months old start to get a little chewy, but are still relatively soft.

The shell surrounding the meat and water also hardens with age. The younger coconuts have a relatively soft shell that is easy to penetrate. As the coconut matures, the shell can become very hard. Fully matured coconut shells are so hard you almost need a sledgehammer to open them.

If you have a machete or meat cleaver, you can open the coconut in the traditional way by chopping the top off. The top is the pointed end. The flat end is for resting on the table. If you peel back the husk on the bottom of the coconut, you will discover the three "eyes." When

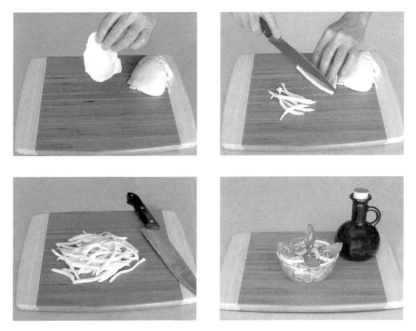

Spoon the meat out of the shell in as large chunks as possible. Lay the coconut out on a cutting board. Cut the coconut into thin strips. Use just as you would cooked pasta.

you open a mature coconut, you first puncture one of the eyes and drain the liquid. However, with a young coconut, you open the opposite end to access the liquid and the meat.

If you are not handy with a machete, you can cut the end off the coconut with a large kitchen knife. A serrated knife works best as you will need to use a sawing motion to cut through the shell. The shell isn't that difficult to cut. It's kind of like slicing a hard loaf of bread.

After consuming the water, don't throw the shell away just yet. Spoon out and eat the delicious meat inside. If the hole in the coconut is too small, simply cut a larger one. The meat comes out with little effort.

Young coconut meat is very tender, with a gelatin-like texture and mild sweet flavor. Its texture and flavor somewhat resembles cooked pasta. For this reason, you can use young coconut meat to make coconut pasta. Coconut pasta can be used just like any other pasta to make spaghetti or pasta salads. Young coconut meat cut into cubes or strips can be added to fruit and vegetable salads. Its mild sweetness makes it a suitable complement to both fruits and vegetables. It is even tasty roasted on a grill.

COCONUT TODDY

If you are in the tropics you will encounter another coconut beverage that is very similar to coconut water. In the Philippines it is called coconut toddy or tuba. It is also sometimes referred to as "coconut juice" and looks and tastes somewhat similar to coconut water. In Latin America it is sold on the streets as coconut juice. It is very sweet and generally served chilled with a scoop of roasted peanuts on top. It is delicious and the nuts are a pleasant addition to the drink.

Coconut toddy is tree sap from a coconut palm. It is somewhat similar to coconut water but has a higher sugar content. Sap is collected from the cut end of the stem in which the flower grows and what would eventually develop into a bunch of coconuts. It is harvested twice daily. Workers climb the tree morning and evening to gather the sap that collects in containers placed under the oozing end of cut flower stems.

Depending on when the toddy was collected, it may be at some stage of fermentation, which gives it a little effervescence, kind of like soda. If you don't live in the tropics, you are not likely to find toddy, at least not fresh, unfermented toddy. Because of its high sugar content, it ferments extremely quickly.

Coconut water and toddy look alike. Since they are both often referred to as "coconut juice," the term can cause confusion. You can tell the difference between the two by the way they are sold. Fresh coconut water is served inside a whole coconut. The coconut serves as the container. It is chopped open and a straw is inserted. Coconut toddy, on the other hand, is served in a glass and comes from a jug or barrel. It is much sweeter than coconut water and often slightly fermented.

Because of the high sugar content of the toddy, it is used to make palm or coconut sugar. To make the sugar the toddy is boiled down into a syrup and crystallized to form sugar. The sugar has a sweet molasses-like taste.

Coconut toddy is often allowed to ferment into a sort of coconut wine, which is slightly alcoholic due to yeast fermentation. The fermented toddy can be distilled to increase the alcohol content, producing a coconut gin.

Note to Readers

Coconut water is helping many people enjoy a better level of health and fitness. I would like to know how coconut water is helping you. Please write and share your successes, experiences, recipes, and ideas with me. You can write to me in care of The Coconut Research Center, PO Box 25203, Colorado Springs, Colorado 80936, USA or email me at bruce@coconutresearchcenter.org. For more information about coconut, diet, and health ask for a free copy/subscription to my *Healthy Ways Newsletter*.

10

Coconut Water Recipes

Coconut water is delicious just as it is straight from the coconut. However, coconut water can be used in making a variety of beverages and foods. This chapter provides several examples of how coconut water can be used in food preparation. Most of these recipes are very simple and easy to make.

Coconut water and coconut milk go well together. A number of the recipes in this chapter call for the use of coconut milk. You can use canned or fresh coconut milk. Canned coconut milk can be found in almost every grocery store. It is usually sold in the Asian foods section. Look for a brand that does not have preservatives. You can also make your own coconut milk from fresh *mature* coconuts—the brown hairy coconuts sold at all grocery stores. Fresh coconut milk is delicious and is superior to the canned variety; however, it does take a bit of effort to make. Directions for making your own coconut milk are found at the end of this chapter.

For readers who prefer to use metric measurements, please refer to the following conversions for the recipes in this chapter.

1 teaspoon = 5 ml	½ cup = 120 ml
1 tablespoon = 15 ml	¾ cup =180 ml
¼ cup = 60 ml	1 cup = 240 ml

Additional coconut water recipes can be found online at www.piccadillybooks.com.

COCONUT ICE

Coconut ice is a very simple and tasty, refreshing treat, especially in the summer. All you have to do is freeze coconut water. That's it. Pour the water into an ice cube tray and put into the freezer. To make a coconut water slushy, put the frozen ice cubes in a blender and blend until smooth. To make coconut water popsicles, insert a popsicle stick into each cube after the water has been in the freezer for about an hour and is starting to crystallize. Let the water continue to freeze until hard. Remove and eat like a popsicle.

COCONUT LIME DRINK

You've heard the lyrics of the Harry Belafonte song "Put the lime in the coconut and drink it all up..." Lime and coconut water is a popular combination in the islands. Rum is sometimes added, but we will leave it out of our version. The important thing to keep in mind when making this recipe is that you are *not* making limeade. You are just giving the coconut water a hint of lime flavor. The recipe is very simple, all you do is add a few drops (8-12) of fresh lime juice to a glass of coconut water, stir, and enjoy.

COCONUT KEFIR WITH LIME

This is a delicious drink made from coconut water kefir. Make the coconut water kefir described in Chapter 7. Add about 5-6 drops of fresh lime juice per cup.

COCONUT WATER SODA

½ cup coconut water
½ cup carbonated water
1 tablespoon frozen concentrated fruit juice

This recipe produces a carbonated like fruity coconut juice drink. Simply combine all three ingredients. Use any type of frozen juice concentrate for the flavoring like apple juice, grape juice, or mango kiwi juice. Do not reconstitute before adding to the other ingredients.

COCONUT CIDER
This recipe produces a delightful drink with a bit of a kick. The nuts add to the enjoyment.

1 cup coconut water
1½ teaspoons apple cider vinegar
1 tablespoon roasted salted peanuts or pecans (optional)

Combine coconut water and vinegar and stir. Top with nuts. For a milder flavor, use just 1 teaspoon of vinegar.

NON-DAIRY MILK
This recipe makes a wonderful replacement for dairy milk. It tastes good straight from the glass or can be used on cereal or in almost any recipe calling for milk.

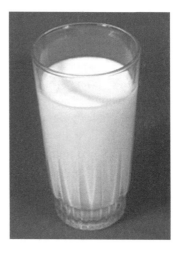

½ cup coconut milk
1 cup coconut water
Pinch sea salt

Combine all ingredients, stir, and chill. Serve cold.

NON-DAIRY STRAWBERRY MILK
Make the Non-Dairy Milk described above and combine it with 1 cup of fresh strawberries in a blender. Blend until smooth.

HOT COCOA

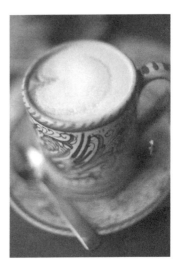

½ cup coconut water
½ cup coconut milk
1 tablespoon powdered cocoa
1 tablespoon sugar
⅛ teaspoon vanilla

Combine all ingredients except for the vanilla into a saucepan and place on medium heat on stove. Heat and stir until all ingredients are blended and texture is uniform. Remove from heat and add vanilla. Serve warm.

YOUNG COCONUT SMOOTHIE

This is a very simple, but delicious recipe. It's surprising how tasty it is. You need one whole young coconut. Open it and drain out the liquid and set it aside. Scoop out all of the soft coconut meat. Portions of the tan colored shell lining will cling to the meat, which is okay; just be certain to remove any large woody pieces—but you don't need to bother removing all of it. Combine all of the meat and coconut water into a blender. Blend until the mixture turns milky white, and coconut chunks are finely chopped. Drink and enjoy. The small bits of coconut add to the pleasure of this drink.

CREAMY FRUIT SMOOTHIE

This recipe makes an all natural, mildly sweet fruit smoothie. You can use any fruit or combination of fruits of your choice. Berries and tropical fruits are excellent choices.

1 cup coconut milk or yogurt
1 cup coconut water
3 cups chopped fruit

186

Chill ingredients beforehand. You can even freeze the coconut water and fruit for a thick smoothie. Combine all ingredients and mix in a blender until smooth. Enjoy immediately or put into the freezer to thicken. Stevia or another sweetener can be added if desired.

CREAMY MANGO SMOOTHIE

1 cup coconut water
½ cup coconut milk
¾ cup pineapple, chopped
1 cup mango, chopped

Chill ingredients beforehand. Combine all ingredients and mix in a blender until smooth.

TROPICAL FRUIT SMOOTHIE

1½ cups coconut water
½ banana
1½ cups pineapple
1 mango
¼ cup shredded coconut

Chill ingredients beforehand. Combine all ingredients and mix in a blender until smooth.

PINA COLADA SMOOTHIE

1 cup coconut water
½ cup coconut milk
2 cups pineapple

Combine all ingredients and mix in a blender until smooth.

BANANA BERRY SMOOTHIE

1½ cups coconut water
¾ cup coconut milk
1 banana
2 cups mixed berries
1 tablespoon honey (optional)

Chill ingredients beforehand. Combine all ingredients and mix in a blender until smooth.

STRAWBERRY SMOOTHIE

½ cup coconut milk
1 cup coconut water
1½ cups strawberries
1 teaspoon honey (optional)

Combine all ingredients into a blender and blend.

COCONUT TEA

Coconut water makes an excellent base for herbal teas. All you do is replace the water you would normally use with coconut water. Heat 1 cup of coconut water to boiling, remove from heat, and seep the teabag in the hot water for 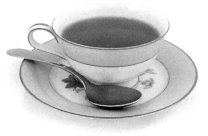 about 5 minutes. You can use almost any type of herbal tea. Once you start using coconut water for your tea, you won't want to go back to using plain water again.

GRAPEFRUIT DRINK

This is a nice blend of fresh grapefruit juice and coconut water. The coconut water gives some sweetness to the otherwise normally tart grapefruit juice. The formula is simple: combine 1 part fresh grapefruit juice with two parts coconut water. To make a 12 ounce drink (1½ cups), mix ½ cup of grapefruit juice with 1 cup of coconut water.

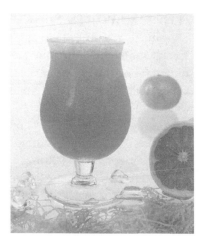

COCONUT VEGGIE JUICE MIX

Fresh vegetable juices are often overpowering unless they are diluted with water or fruit juice. Coconut water makes a nice medium to mellow out the strong flavor of pure vegetable juices. Combine 2-4 parts coconut water with 1 part vegetable juice. The exact amount of coconut water needed will vary depending on the type of vegetable juice. Strong flavored vegetables will require more coconut water. Below are some examples.

Coconut Beet Juice

Combine 2 parts coconut water with 1 part beet juice.

Carrot Beet Juice

Combine 4 parts coconut water with 1 part beet juice and 1 part carrot juice.

Coconut Fruit and Vegetable Juice

Adding some fruit juice enhances the flavor quite a bit. Combine 2 parts coconut water with 1 part fruit juice (apple, orange, grape, etc.) and 1 part vegetable juice.

VITAMIN SPORTS PUNCH

This recipe produces a slightly fizzy vitamin packed fruit punch. Because of the high vitamin and mineral content, including 60 mg of sodium (as sodium bicarbonate), this recipe makes an excellent sports rehydration drink. Combine one glass (about 12 ounces) of coconut water with one 3-ounce packet of Emergen-C powdered fruit mix, stir, and enjoy. Emergen-C is a super energy booster dietary supplement containing 32 vitamin and mineral complexes in a fruit flavored base. One packet contains 1000 mg of vitamin C. Emergen-C comes in a variety of flavors including lemon lime, tropical punch, tangerine, black cherry, raspberry, and acai berry. Emergen-C is available in the vitamin section of most grocery and health food stores.

FRUIT SOUP

You can make a variety of refreshing, mostly raw soups using coconut water as the soup "stock" combined with fresh fruits and other ingredients. Serve it in a bowl with a spoon or drink it from a mug like you would any soup. In addition to coconut water, you can also use kefir or lacto-fermented coconut water or coconut tea as the soup base. There is a lot of room for experimentation here. Try combining different teas and tea blends with various fruits. Below are some examples. Directions for making the soups are simple, just combine all the ingredients and enjoy. Most of these soups taste best chilled. Chill ingredients before combining. If you are using a tea soup base, cool it down before adding other ingredients.

Coconut Blueberry Soup

    1½ cups coconut water
    ½ cup young coconut meat, finely chopped
    ½ cup blueberries

Berry Good Soup

    1 cup coconut water*
    ½ apple, finely chopped
    1 cup berries (strawberries, blueberries, raspberries, or boysenberries)

1 tablespoon pecans

*This recipe also tastes great using lacto-fermented coconut water or ginger tea.

Tropical Fruit Soup
2 cups coconut water
1 banana, cut into small pieces
1 mango, cut into small pieces
1 cup pineapple, cut into small pieces
¼ cup shredded dried coconut

Melon Soup
1 cup coconut water*
1 cup watermelon, cut into bite-size pieces
½ cup cantaloupe, cut into bite-size pieces
½ cup honeydew, cut into bite-size piece.

*You can also use kefir or lacto-fermented coconut water or ginger tea. Fermented coconut water adds a delightful fizz to this soup.

Apple Cinnamon Soup
1 cup cinnamon coconut water tea*
1 apple, diced
¼ cup raisins
¼ cup, pecans, chopped

*You can make this tea with just cinnamon or you can use a commercial blend such as Celestial Seasonings Sugar Plum Spice tea which is a combination of hibiscus, roasted barley, roasted chicory, rosehips, chamomile, cinnamon, ginger, and other spices.

COCONUT RICE
Coconut water can make a nice substitute for water in preparing rice dishes.

½ cup brown rice
1¼ cups coconut water
½ cup shredded coconut
Dash sea salt
2 teaspoons honey
½ cup coconut milk
¼ cup slivered almonds, toasted (optional)

Soak the rice in coconut water in a saucepan for at least 4 hours. Stir in coconut and salt; bring to a boil, reduce heat, cover, and simmer for 60 minutes or until rice is tender. (If rice is not soaked beforehand, you will need to cook it for at least 90 minutes.) Remove from heat, stir in honey and coconut milk. Top with slivered almonds. Serve hot. Makes 2 servings.

APPLE CINNAMON RICE

This is a flavorful mildly sweet rice dish made with coconut water.

½ cup brown rice
1 cup plus 1 tablespoon coconut water
½ apple, chopped
2 tablespoons raisins
1 teaspoon cinnamon
⅛ teaspoon nutmeg
Dash sea salt
1 teaspoon honey
½ cup coconut milk

Soak the rice in coconut water in a saucepan for at least 4 hours. Stir in raisins, cinnamon, nutmeg, and salt; bring to a boil, reduce heat, cover, and simmer for 60 minutes or until rice is tender. (If rice is not soaked beforehand, you will need to cook it for at least 90 minutes.) Remove from heat, stir in honey and coconut milk. Serve hot. Makes 2 servings.

ORANGE CARDAMOM RICE
This is a delightfully flavorful rice dish.

½ cup brown rice
1 cup coconut water
½ teaspoon cardamom
Dash sea salt
½ orange, pealed and sliced
1 teaspoon honey
½ cup coconut milk

Soak the rice in coconut water in a saucepan for at least 4 hours. Stir in cardamom and salt; bring to a boil, reduce heat, cover, and simmer for 60 minutes or until rice is tender. (If rice is not soaked beforehand, you will need to cook it for at least 90 minutes.) Peel orange, separate into sections, and cut into several pieces. Mix orange pieces, honey, and milk into rice. Serve hot.

WHOLE WHEAT PANCAKES

1 cup whole wheat flour
½ teaspoon sea salt
1 teaspoon baking powder
1 cup coconut water
2 tablespoons oil

Mix flour, salt, baking powder together in a bowl. Put oil in a skillet, heat slightly, and coat pan surface. Pour the excess oil into the dry ingredients and stir in coconut water. Spoon batter onto to skillet making pancakes about 3 inches in diameter. Cook until puffed and edges become dry. Turn and cook the other side. Makes about 9 pancakes. Serve topped with your choice of syrup or fruit.

Blueberry Pancakes
Follow the directions for making Whole Wheat Pancakes and fold into the finished batter ½ cup of fresh blueberries. Cook as directed.

Banana Pancakes

Follow the directions for making Whole Wheat Pancakes. Cut 1 banana into several slices and then cut each slice into quarters. Fold banana pieces into batter. Cook as directed.

Coconut Pineapple Pancakes

Follow the directions for making Whole Wheat Pancakes. Add ¼ cup of shredded coconut to dry ingredients and fold into finished batter ½ cup chopped pineapple. Cook as directed.

CHOCOLATE PANCAKES

These pancakes taste so good it's almost a sin.

1 cup whole wheat flour
2½ tablespoons cocoa powder
½ teaspoon sea salt
1 teaspoon baking powder
1 cup coconut water
½ cup coconut milk
1 tablespoon oil

Mix flour, cocoa, salt, baking powder together in a bowl. Stir in coconut water and coconut milk until batter is smooth. Heat oil in a skillet and coat bottom of pan. Spoon batter onto skillet making pancakes about 3 inches in diameter. Cook until puffed and edges become dry. Turn and cook the other side. Makes 10-12 pancakes. Serve with your choice of topping.

COCO BANANACAKES

This is an absolutely delicious novelty pancake.

1 cup whole wheat flour
2½ tablespoons cocoa powder
½ teaspoon sea salt
1 teaspoon baking powder

1 cup coconut water
½ cup coconut milk
1 banana, sliced and quartered
1 tablespoon oil

Mix flour, cocoa, salt, baking powder together in a bowl. Stir in coconut water and coconut milk until batter is smooth. Cut 1 banana into several slices and then cut each slice into quarters. Fold banana pieces into batter. Heat oil in a skillet and coat bottom of pan. Spoon batter onto skillet making pancakes about 3 inches in diameter. Cook until puffed and edges become dry. Turn and cook the other side. Makes about 12 pancakes. Serve with your choice of topping.

Double Coco Bananacakes

Coconut and chocolate make excellent partners. This recipe doubles up on the coconut content by adding coconut meat. Follow the directions for making Coco Bananacakes and add ½ cup of shredded coconut to dry ingredients. Cook as directed.

HOW TO MAKE COCONUT MILK

Coconut milk is made by squeezing shredded coconut meat along with a little water, producing in a rich creamy beverage that looks very much like cow's milk. Coconut milk looks and tastes very different from coconut water. It has a high fat content which gives it a creamy texture. If allowed to sit for any length of time, the oil rich cream tends to separate and float to the top. This is referred to as coconut cream. Sometimes this cream is scooped off to make deserts. The lower portion is more watery. If you store the milk in the refrigerator, it will separate. To remix it, simply shake or stir it up before using. Most commercially produced coconut milk has thickeners added to prevent or reduce separation.

Coconut milk is not sweet unless it has sugar added so it can be used as a cream base in soups, curries, and other non-sweet dishes. Of course, with a little sweetening, it tastes great in smoothies, beverages, and desserts.

Coconut milk can be made at home from fresh mature coconuts. Mature coconuts have the greatest amount of oil, which is needed to make coconut milk. You cannot make coconut milk from young coconuts because they lack sufficient meat and oil.

You can make coconut milk in one of two ways—from fresh coconuts or from dried shredded coconut. Both ways are described below.

Coconut Milk from Fresh Coconut

Pierce two eyes of a coconut. An ice pick works well. One eye is very soft. The other two are a little more difficult to penetrate. Use one hole to pour out the water; the other hole is made to equalize air pressure so the water will easily come out of the first opening. Drain the liquid.

Crack open the coconut and remove the white meat. The shell is very hard so you will need a hammer. Place the coconut on a hard surface, such as a cement floor, when you hit it with the hammer. Break it into several pieces. Pry the meat off with a knife. An alternate way to remove the meat is to put the drained coconut into a preheated oven at 325 degrees F (165 C) for 30 minutes. Heating makes it easier to crack the shell open and remove the meat.

The meat will have a thin brown layer where it was attached to the shell. You do not need to remove this layer. Cut the meat into small pieces. Place the meat into a blender along with just enough hot water to cover the coconut. The less water you use, the creamier the resulting milk will be. Blend until the coconut is finely chopped.

Place several layers of cheesecloth in a strainer. Pour the coconut mixture through the cheesecloth and strainer, collecting the liquid in a bowl. Wrap the cheesecloth around the shredded coconut, and with your hands squeeze as much of the liquid out of the meat as possible. This is your first squeezing or pressing. The resulting liquid is very rich and creamy. If you like, you can put the coconut back into the blender with a little more hot water and repeat the process to extract a little more milk. The second pressing will yield a slightly less rich milk.

Discard the shredded coconut. Use the milk immediately or store in the refrigerator. Use the milk within three days.

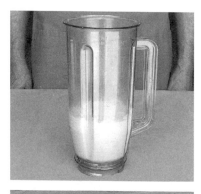

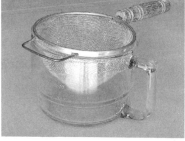

Blend coconut meat and hot water in a blender.

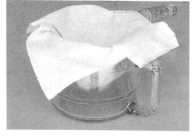

Put a strainer over a bowl to catch the milk.

Place several layers of cheese cloth or some other fabric over the strainer.

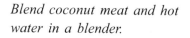

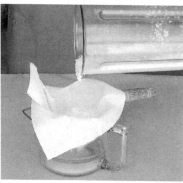

Pour the coconut mixture into the strainer.

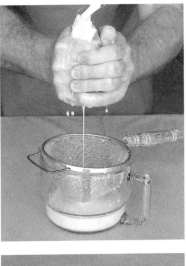

Squeeze all the liquid out of the shredded meat inside the cloth.

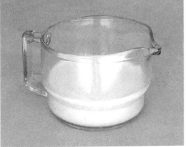

The coconut milk is finished. Drink it warm or place into the refrigerator to chill.

Coconut Milk from Dried Coconut

Empty an 8 ounce package of unsweetened, unsulfured shredded coconut into a blender. Add 1 cup of hot water. Blend for about 30 seconds and allow the mixture a few minutes to cool.

Place several layers of cheesecloth in a strainer. Pour the coconut mixture through the cheesecloth and strainer, collecting the liquid in a bowl. Wrap the cheesecloth around the shredded coconut and with your hands squeeze as much of the liquid out of the meat as possible. This is your first squeezing or pressing. You can put the coconut back into the blender with a little more hot water and repeat the process to extract a little more milk.

Discard the coconut and store the coconut milk in the refrigerator. Use within three days.

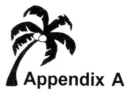

Appendix A

Guide to Giving Oral Rehydration Therapy at Home

The two most important treatments for diarrhea are oral rehydration therapy (ORT) and continued feeding. When ORT is going on, for diarrhea, feeding should continue. The two go hand in hand. A child may survive acute diarrhea, but then die from the consequences of malnutrition. Not giving any food for 48 hours used to be the standard recommendation. We now know better; continued feeding results in faster recovery and better nourished children.

ORT should be started as soon as diarrhea begins in order to prevent dehydration. Any delay may mean the child's condition gets worse. A dehydrated child is usually thirsty and will want to drink the rehydration fluid.

Vomiting itself does not mean that oral rehydration cannot be given, although it is best not to give solid food until the child can keep it down. As long as more fluid enters than exits, rehydration will be accomplished. It is only when the volume of fluid and electrolyte loss in vomit and stool exceeds what is taken in that dehydration will continue.

It should be emphasized that oral rehydration does *not* stop diarrhea. Although ORT prevents dehydration it does not reduce the volume, frequency or the duration of diarrhea. It keeps the body hydrated and free from the discomforting symptoms and danger of dehydration until the diarrhea passes. Diarrhea will continue until it has run its course.

The information in this section is adapted from *Dialogue on Diarrhoea* 1993;52:7

199

Rehydration Fluid

The World Health Organization recommends commercial Oral Rehydration Salt (ORS) solution if available. Other acceptable drinks include green coconut water, water in which a cereal (such as rice) has been cooked, unsweetened fresh fruit juice, water with ½ teaspoon salt and 4 teaspoons sugar per liter. For moderate and severe cases of dehydration commercial sports drinks should be avoided, especially in younger children as these solutions contain too much sugar and not enough electrolytes.

How to Give ORT

Oral rehydration fluids can be given in the following ways: by cup, spoon, or dripper (for small infants). The spoon is the best method for most infants and young children because it allows fluid to be given at a steady rate in small amounts, which reduces vomiting.

A cup may be used for children older than five years and for adults. Very small babies should be given rehydration fluid with a spoon or a plastic dropper. The mother should insert the dropper between the cheek and teeth and the contents should be gently squeezed at a rate of 1 teaspoon (5 ml) every 3-4 minutes. Droppers should be cleaned thoroughly after every use.

Babies should not be given fluid too quickly as they might vomit or choke. Feeding bottles should not be used as they are difficult to clean and the rate of flow of the fluid cannot be controlled.

Be patient and persistent when giving fluid. If a child refuses to drink, it usually means that enough fluid has been given.

Continue to Feed the Child

Continue the child's normal diet. Give small meals frequently, at least six times a day. If possible, give a food that contains salt.

How Often

Rehydration fluid should be given at a steady rate in small amounts. One teaspoonful every 2-3 minutes is a useful guide (see below for amounts according to age). This allows time for it to be absorbed and reduces the risk of vomiting.

How Much

The amount of rehydration fluid given should be about the same as the volume of vomit and stool passed. However, it may not always be possible to accurately measure the volume lost, so guidelines are as follows:

= A child under two years old should be given about ¼ - ½ cup (60-120ml) of rehydration fluid after each loose stool.

= Older children will require ½ - 1 cup (120-240ml).

= Children over ten years old and adults can take as much as they want.

If a child is usually breastfed, continue breastfeeding in between giving oral rehydration fluid.

It is important to emphasize giving plenty of rehydration fluid. The mother should be advised that just giving a few sips of rehydration fluid is not enough; the amounts described earlier should be given until diarrhea stops.

If the child has many watery stools, vomits repeatedly, is very thirsty, or is eating or drinking poorly, he or she should be taken to the nearest health center. The child should also be taken if there is fever or blood in the stool.

Rehydration is generally adequate when the child no longer feels thirsty and has a normal urine output. Once the child is rehydrated and nausea passes normal eating normal eating may resume.

Potential Problems

If the child is vomiting, ORT should not be stopped. Instead, the mother should wait for five to ten minutes, then continue giving the solution but more slowly, a teaspoonful every 3-4 minutes.

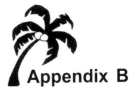

Appendix B

Resources

USEFUL WEBSITES

Coconut Research Center

www.coconutresearchcenter.org
The Coconut Research Center is a nonprofit organization dedicated to educating the medical community and general public about the health aspects of coconut and related products. This website contains numerous articles, current research, nutritional information, resources for educational materials and products, and includes an open discussion forum. A free subscription to the *Healthy Ways Newsletter* is available on request. Contact bruce@coconutresearchcenter.org.

Piccadilly Books, Ltd.

www.piccadillybooks.com.
This website lists the best books and tapes currently available on the health aspects of coconut and related products. Call or write and ask for a free catalog: Piccadilly Books, Ltd. P.O. Box 25203, Colorado Springs, CO 80936, USA, phone 719-550-9887, email info@piccadillybooks.com.

Global Health Solutions, Inc.

www.watercure.com

This website was created by F. Batmanghelidj, MD the author of *Your Body's Many Cries for Water*. It offers books, tapes, and education about the body's need for water and the medical conditions associated with chronic dehydration.

Body Ecology
www.bodyecology.com
This website provides information and products for a healthy digestive system. The philosophy behind the Body Ecology Diet is to balance the organisms living within the digestive tract using probiotics and foods that support healthy digestive function.

Puriti Programs for Life, Ltd.
www.puriti.org
Puriti has designed a set of detoxification programs based on the use of coconut water and includes fruit and vegetable juices along with other coconut products and cleansing herbs. The detox programs range from 1 to 8 days. These programs are being used in many health spas and resorts in Asia, where they were originally developed. The programs are also available through this website.

BIBLIOGRAPHY

Coconut Cures: Preventing and Treating Common Health Problems with Coconut, Bruce Fife, 2005: Piccadilly Books, Ltd., Colorado Springs, CO.

The Coconut Oil Miracle, 4th Ed. Bruce Fife, 2004: Avery, New York, NY.

The Coconut Odyssey: The Bounteous Possibilities of the Tree of Life, Mike Foale, 2003: Australian Centre for International Agricultural Research, Canberra, ACT.

Your Body's Many Cries for Water, 2nd Ed. F. Batmanghelidj, 1997: Global Health Solutions, Inc., Falls Church, VA.

The Body Ecology Diet, 9th Ed. Donna Gates, 2006: Body Ecology, Decatur, GA.

The Healing Crisis, 2nd Ed., Bruce Fife, 2002: Piccadilly Books, Ltd., Colordo Springs, CO.

Seasalt's Hidden Powers, Jacques de Langre, 1994: Happiness Press, Asheville, NC.

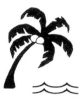

References

Chapter 1: Living Water From the Tree of Life
1. Bustamante, J.O. New Biotechnological applications of coconuts. *Electronic Journal of Biotechnology* 2004;7:1-4.

Chapter 2: The Intravenous Use of Coconut Water
1. Hicking, A. Coconut water, its potential as a natural parenteral fluid, Tenth Pacific Science Congress, Honolulu, Hawaii, Aug. 21-Sept.6, 1961.
2. Jelliffe, D.B. Coconut milk infusion. Letters to the Editor. *Lancet* 1966;2:968.
3. Olurin, E.O., et al. Intravenous coconut water therapy in surgical practice. *WAMJ* 1972;21:124-131.
4. Campbell-Falck, D., et al. The intravenous use of coconut water. *Am J Emerg Med* 2000;18:108-111.
5. Pradera, E.S., et al. Coconut water: clinical and experimental study. *Amer J Dis Child* 1942;64:977.
6. Goldsmith, H.S. Coconut water for intravenous therapy. *Brit J Surg* 1962;49:421-422.
7. Ciro, B.J. and Dreiss, G. Renal secretion in man. *Arch Hosp Rosales, San Salvador* 1943;35:66.
8. Mojumdar, N.G. Intravenous use of green coconut water in pediatric practice; a preliminary report. *J Indian Med Assoc* 1951;20:211-212.

9. Eiseman, B., et al. Use of coconut water of intravenous infusion. *J M A Thailand* 1952;35:29.

10. Eiseman, B. Intravenous infusion of coconut water. *AMA Archives of Surgery* 1954;68:167-178.

11. Goldsmith, H.S. Coco-nut water for intravenous therapy. *Br J Surg* 1962;49:421-422.

12. Carpenter, C.C., et al. Green coconut water: a readily available source of potassium for the cholera patient. *Bull Calcutta Sch Trop Med* 1964;12:20-21.

13. Acharya, V.N., et al. Comparative study of intravenous use of natural coconut water, synthetic coconut water and glucose saline in acute gastro-enteritis. *Indian J Med Res* 1965;53:1069-1073.

14. Ranti, I.S., et al. Coconut water for intravenous fluid therapy. *Paediatr Indones* 1965;5 Suppl:782-792.

15. Rao, P.S., et al. Intravenous administration of coconut water. *J Assoc Physicians India* 1972;20:235-239.

16. Olurin, E.O., et al. Intravenous coconut water therapy in surgical practice. *West Afr Med J* 1972;21:124-131.

17. Anzaldo, F.E. Chemical composition of coconut water as related to its use in intravenous therapy. *Science Review* 1973;14:10-16.

18. Anzaldo, F.E., et al. Coconut water as intravenous fluid. *Philipp J Pediatr* 1975;24:143-166.

19. Lqbal, Q.M. Direct infusion of coconut water. *Med J Malaysia* 1976;30:221-223.

20. Kuberski, T. Coconut water as a rehydration fluid. *N Z Med J* 1979;90:98-100.

21. Pummer, S., et al. Influence of coconut water on hemostasis. *Am J Emerg Med* 2001;19:287-289.

22. Mantena, S.K., et al. In vitro evaluation of antioxidant properties of Cocos nucifera Linn. Water. *Die Nahrung* 2003;47:126-131.

23. Goldsmith, H.S. Coconut water for intravenous therapy. *Brit J Surg* 1962;49:421-422.

24. Campbell-Falck, D. et al. The intravenous use of coconut water. *Am J Emerg Med* 2000;18:108-111.

25. Fife, B. *Coconut Cures: Preventing and Treating Common Health Problems with Coconut.* Colorado Springs, Colorado: Piccadilly Books. 2005.

26. Olurin, E.O., et al. Intravenous coconut water therapy in surgical practice. *West Afr Med J* 1972;21:124-131.

27. Ibid.

28. Recio, P.M., et al. The intravenous use of coconut water. *Philipp J Surg Spec* 1974;30:119-140.

29. Rao, P.S., et al. Intravenous administration of coconut water. *J Assoc Physicians India* 1972;20:235-239.

30. Eiseman, B., et al. Clinical experience in intravenous administration of coconut water. *AMA Archives of Surgery* 1954;69:87-93.

31. Anzaldo, F.E. Coconut water for intravenous therapy and oral rehydration. *Coconuts Today* 1987;5:108-113.

Chapter 3: Oral Rehydration

1. Kleiner, S.M. Water: an essential but overlooked nutrient. *American Dietetic Association Journal* 1999:99:200-206.

2. Ikpatt, N.W. and Young, M.U. Preliminary study on the attitude of people in two states of Nigeria on diarrhoeal disease and its management. *East Afr Med J* 1992;69:219-222.

3. Harun, N., et al. The use of young coconut water in pediatric cholera, *Pediatr Indonesia* 1979;19:219-225.

4. Ludan, A.C., et al. Modified coconut water for oral rehydration. *Philipp J Pediatr* 1980;29:344-351.

5. Chavalittamrong, B., et al. Electrolytes, sugar, calories, osmolarity and pH of beverages and coconut water. *Southeast Asian J Trop Med Public Health* 1982;13:427-431.

6. Kuberski, T., et al. Coconut water as a rehydration fluid. *N Z Med J* 1979;90:98-100.

7. Anzaldo, F.E., et al. Modified coconut water: a suitable fluid for oral rehydration. *Philippine Journal of Science* 1980;9-14.

8. Rolston, D.D., et al. Food-based solutions are a viable alternative to glucose-electrolyte solutions for oral hydration in acute diarrhoea—studies in a rat model of secretory diarrhoea. *Trans R Soc Trop Med Hyg* 1990;84:156-159.

9. Adams, W. and Bratt, D.E. Young coconut water for home rehydration in children with mild gastroenteritis. *Trop Geogr Med* 1992;44:149-153.

10. Fagundes, N.U., et al. Negative findings for use of coconut water as an oral rehydration solution in childhood diarrhea. *J Am Coll Nutr* 1993;12:190-193.

11. Cooper, E.S. Coconut water. *Lancet* 1986;2:281.

12. International Study Group on Reduced-Osmolarity ORS Solutions. Multicentre evaluation of reduced-osmolarity oral rehydration salts solution. *Lancet* 1995;345:282-285.

13. http://www.fao.org/AG/magazine/0701sp1.htm.

14. Anonymous. Nutrition. You can break the diarrhoea circle. *Afr Women Health* 1993;1:28-29.

15. Sett, A. and Mitra, U. Answers to questions in relation to oral rehydration therapy. *Indian J Public Health* 1994;38:87-88.

16. Anonymous. All about diarrhoea. *Cent Call* 1998;33:12-13.

17. Saat, M., et al. Rehydration after exercise with fresh young coconut water, carbohydrate-electrolyte beverage and plain water. *J Physiol Anthropol* 2002;21:93-104.

18. Shirreffs. S.M. and Maughan, R.J. Rehydration and recovery of fluid balance after exercise. *Exercise and Sport Sciences Reviews* 2000;28:27-32.

19. Maughan, R.J., et al. Post-exercise rehydration in man; effects of electrolyte addition to ingested fluids. *Eur J Appl Phsiol* 1994;69:209-215.

20. Yawata, T. Effect of potassium solution on rehydration in rats: comparison with sodium solution and water. *Jpn J Physiol* 1990;40:369-338.

21. Horowitz, G.Z. Bromism from excessive cola consumption. *Journal of Toxicology* 1997;35:315-320.

Chapter 4: Electrolyte Up Your Life

1. Cohen, H.W. and Alderman, M.H. Sodium, blood pressure, and cardiovascular disease. *Current Opinion in Cardiology* 2007;22:306-310.

2. Whitney, E.N., et al. *Understanding Normal and Clinical Nutrition, 3rd Ed.* St. Paul, MN: West Publishing Company. 1991.

3. Altschul, A.M. and Grommet, J.K. Sodium intake and sodium sensitivity. *Nutrition Reviews* 1980;38:393-402.

4. Rodale, J.I., et al. *Complete Book of Minerals for Health.* Emmaus, PA: Rodale Books. 1970.

5. Adrogue, H.J. and Madias, N.E. Sodium and potassium in the pathogenesis of hypertension. *New Engl J Med* 2007;356:1966-1978.

6. Addison, W.L.T. The use of sodium chloride, potassium chloride, sodium bromide and potassium bromide in cases of arterial hypertension which are amenable to potassium chloride. *Can Med Assoc J* 1928;18:281-285.

7. Krishna, G.G., et al. Increased blood pressure during potassium depletion in normotensive men. *N Engl J Med* 1989;320:117-1182.

8. Anonymous. Supplemental dietary potassium reduced the need for antihypertensive drug therapy. *Nutrition Reviews* 1992;50:144-145.

9. Appel, L.J., et al. A clinical trial of the effects of dietary patterns on blood pressure. *New Engl J Med* 1997;336:1117-1124.

10. Whelton, P.K., et al. Effects of oral potassium on blood pressure. *JAMA* 1997;277:1624-1632.

11. Young, D.B. and McCabe, R.D. Potassium's cardiovascular protective mechanism. *Am J Physiol* 1995;268:R825-R837.

12. Young, D.B. and Ma, G. Vascular protection effects of potassium. *Semin Nephrol* 1999;19:477-486.

13. Prioreschi, P. Experimental cardiac necrosis and potassium. *Canad Med Assoc J* 1967;96:1221-1223.

14. Sasaki S, Zhang XH, Kesteloot H. Dietary sodium, potassium, saturated fat, alcohol, and stroke mortality. *Stroke* 1995;26:783–9.

15. Khaw, K.T. and Barrett-Connor, E. Dietary potassium and stroke-associated mortality. A 12-year prospective population study. *N Engl J Med* 1987;316:235–40.

16. Fang, J., et al. Dietary potassium intake and stroke mortality. *Stroke* 2000;31:1532-1537.

17. Bazzano, L.A., et al. Dietary potassium intake and risk of stroke in US men and women: National Health and Nutrition Examination Survey I epidemiologic follow-up study. *Stroke* 2002;32:1473-1480.

18. Ascherio, A., et al. Intake of potassium, magnesium, calcium, and fiber and risk of stroke among US men. *Circulation* 1998;98:1198-1204.

19. Lemann, J. Jr., et al. Potassium causes calcium retention in healthy adults. *J Nutr* 1993;123:1623-1626.

20. Sebastian, A., et al. Improved mineral balance and skeletal metabolism in postmenopausal women treated with potassium bicarbonate. *N Engl J Med* 1994;330:1776-1781.

21. Tucker, K.L., et al. Potassium, magnesium, and fruit and vegetable intakes are associated with greater bone mineral density in elderly men and women. *Am J Clin Nutr* 1999;69:727-736.

22. New, S.A., et al. Dietary influences on bone mass and bone metabolism: further evidence of a positive link between fruit and vegetable consumption and bone health? *Am J Clin Nutr* 2000;71:142-151.

23. LaCelle, P.L., et al. An investigation of total body potassium in patients with rheumatoid arthritis. Proceedings of the Annual Meeting of the American Rheumatism Association. *Arthritis and Rheumatism* 1964;7:321.

24. Costrini, A.M. cardiovascular and metabolic manifestations of heat stroke and severe heat exhaustion. *Am J Med* 1979;66:296-302.

25. Hubbard, R.W., et al. Effect of low-potassium diet on rat exercise hyperthermia and heatstroke mortality. *J Appl Physiol* 1981;51:8-13.

26. Oopik, V., et al. Effect of alkalosis on plasma epinephrine responses to high intensity cycle exercise in humans. *Eur J Appl Physiol* 2002;87:72-77.

27. Lehr, L., et al. Total body potassium depletion and the need for preoperative nutritional support in Crohn's disease. *Ann Surg* 1982;196:709-714.

28. Elliott, P. Salt and blood pressure. In: Izzo, J.L., Jr, Black H.R. Eds. Hypertension primer. 3rd ed. Dallas: American Heart Association/ council on High Blood Pressure Research, 2003;277-279.

29. Whelton, P.K. Potassium and blood pressure. In: Izzo, J.L., Jr, Black, H.R., eds. Hypertension primer, 3rd ed. Dallas: American Heart Association/Council on High Blood Pressure Research, 2003:280-282.

30. *Dietary reference intakes for water, potassium, sodium, chloride, and sulfate.* Washington, DC: National Academies Press, 2005.

31. Cruz-Coke, R, et al. Influence of migration on blood pressure of Easter Islanders. *Lancet* 1964;15:697-699.

32. Ward, R.H., et al. Tokelau Island Migrant Study: effect of migration on the familial aggregation of blood pressure. *Hypertension* 1980;2:I43-I54.

33. http://www.saltinstitute.org/28.html.

34. Elliott, P. Commentary: role of salt intake in the development of high blood pressure. *International Journal of Epidemiology* 2005;34:975-978.

35. Adrogue, H.J. and Madias, N.E. Sodium and potassium in the pathogenesis of hypertension. *N Engl J Med* 2007;356:1966-1978.

36. Tobian, L. et al. Potassium reduces cerebral hemorrhage and death rate in hypertensive rates, even when blood pressure is not lowered. *Hypertension* 1985;7:I110-I114.

37. Morris, R.C., Jr., et al. Normotensive salt sensitivity: effects of race and dietary potassium. *Hypertension* 1999;33:18-23.

38. Alleyne, T., et al. The control of hypertension by use of coconut water and mauby: two tropical food drinks. *West Indian Med J* 2005;54:3-8.

39. A Compilation, *Technical Data Handbook on the Coconut: Its Products and By-Products.* Quezon City, Philippines: Philippine Coconut Authority. 1979.

40. Kuberski, T., et al. Coconut water as a rehydration fluid. *N Z Med J* 1979;90:98-100.

Chapter 5: A Health Tonic

1. Young, D.B. and McCabe, R.D. Potassium's cardiovascular protective mechanism. *Am J Physiol* 1995;268:R825-R837.

2. Macalalag, E.V. and Macalalag, A.L. Bukolysis: young coconut water renoclysis for urinary stone dissolution. *Int Surg* 1987;72:247.

3. Eiseman, B., et al. Clinical experience in intravenous administration of coconut water. *AMA Archives of Surgery* 1954;69:87-93.

4. Eiseman, B., et al. Intravenous infusion of coconut water. *AMA Archives of Surgery* 1954;68:167-178.

5. Zhao, G., et al. Effects of coconut juice on the formation of hyperlipidemia and atherosclerosis. *Chinese Journal of Preventive Medicine* 1995;29:216-218.

6. Sandhya, V.G. and Rajamohan, T. Beneficial effects of coconut water feeding on lipid metabolism in cholesterol-fed rats. *J Med Food* 2006;9:400-407.

7. Alleyne, T., et al. The control of hypertension by use of coconut water and mauby: two tropical food drinks. *West Indian Med J* 2005;54:3-8.

8. The sixth report of the Joint National Committee on prevention, detection, evaluation, and treatment of high blood pressure. *Arch Intern Med.* 1997;157:2413–2446.

9. 1999 World Health Organization–International Society of Hypertension Guidelines for the Management of Hypertension; Guidelines Subcommittee. *J Hypertens.* 1999;17:151–183.

10. Veterans Administration Cooperative Study Group on Antihypertensive Agents. Effects of treatment on morbidity in hypertension. II. Results in patients with diastolic blood pressure averaging 90 through 114 mm Hg. *JAMA.* 1970;213:1143–1152.

11. Messerli FH, Grossman E, and Goldbourt U. Are beta-blockers efficacious as first-line therapy for hypertension in the elderly? A systematic review. *JAMA.* 1998;279:1903–1907.

12. SHEP Cooperative Research Group. Prevention of stroke by antihypertensive drug treatment in older persons with isolated systolic hypertension. Final results of the Systolic Hypertension in the Elderly Program (SHEP). *JAMA* 1991;265:3255-3254.

13. Staessen, J.A., et al. Randomised double-blind comparison of placebo and active treatment for older patients with isolated systolic hypertension. The Systolic Hypertension in Europe (Syst-Eur) Trial Investigators. *Lancet* 1997;350:757-764.

14. Wang, B.Y., et al. Dietary arginine prevents atherogenesis in the coronary artery of the hypercholesterolemic rabbit. *J Am Coll Cardiol* 1994;23:452-458.

15. Cooke, J.P., et al. Antiatherogenic effects of L-arginine in the hypercholesterolemic rabbit. *J Clin Invest* 1992;90:1168-1172.

16. Shah, N.J., et al. Use of coco-nut water in treatment of congestive cardiac failure. *Ind Jour Med Res* 1956;44:341-351.

17. Poblete, G.S., et al. The effect of coconut water on intraocular pressure of normal subjects. *Philipp J Ophthal* 1999;24:3-5.

18. Whelton, P.K., et al. Clinical outcomes in antihypertensive treatment of type 2 diabetes, impaired fasting glucose concentration, and normoglycemia: Antihypertensive and Lipid-Lowering Treatment to Prevent Heart Attack Trial (ALLHAT). *Arch Intern Med* 2005;165:1401-1409.

19. Gannon, M.C., et al. Oral arginine does not stimulate an increase in insulin concentration but delays glucose disposal. *Am J Clin Nutr* 2002;76:1016-1022.

20. Piatti P.M., et al. Long-term oral L-arginine administration improves peripheral aud hepatic insulin sensitivity in type 2 diabetic patients. *Diab Care* 2001;24:875-80.

21. Maxwell, A.J. and Cooke, J.P. Cardiovascular effects of L-arginine. *Current Opinion in Nephrology & Hypertension* 1998;7:63-70.

22. Griffin, N., et al. Topical L-Arginine Gel Lowers Resting Anal Pressure. *Diseases of the Colon & Rectum* 2004;45:1332-1336.

23. Nenoff, P., et al. Topically applied arginine hydrochloride. Effect on urea content of stratum corneum and skin hydration in atopic eczema and skin aging. *Hautarzt* 2004;55:58-64.

Chapter 6: The Youth Solution

1. Van Overbeek, J., et al. Factors in coconut milk essential for growth and development of Datura embryos. *Science* 1941;94:350-351.

2. Kadiri, M., et al. Responses of some Nigerian vegetables of plnat growth regulator treatments. *Rev Biol Trop* 1997;44-45:23-28.

3. Miller, et al. Structure and synthesis of kinetin. *J Am Chem Soc* 1955;78:2662-2663.

4. Ge, L., et al. Identification of kinetin and kinetin riboside in coconut (Cocos nucifera L.) water using a combined approach of liquid chromatography-tandem mass spectrometry, high performance liquid chromatography and capillary electrophoresis. *J Chromatogr B Analyt Technol Biomed Life Sci* 2005;829:26-34.

5. Ge, L., et al. Determination of cytokinins in coconut (Cocos nucifera L.) water using capillary zone electrophoresis-tandem mass spectrometry. *Electrophoresis* 2006;27:2171-2181.

6. Verbeke, P., et al. Kinetin inhibits protein oxidation and glycoxidation in vitro. *Biochem Biophys Res Commun* 2000;276:1265-1270.

7. Barciszewski, J., et al. A mechanism for the in vivo formation of N6-furfuryladenine, kinetin, as a secondary oxidative damage product of DNA 1997;414:457-460.

8. McDaniel, D.H., et al. Idebenone: a new antioxidant – Part 1. Relative assessment of oxidative stress protection capacity compared to commonly known antioxidants. *J Cosmet Dermatol* 2005;4:10-17.

9. Silva, J.R., et al. Effect of coconut water and Braun-Collins solutions at different temperatures and incubation times on the morphology of goat preantral follicles preserved in vitro. *Theriogenology* 2000;54:809-822.

10. Rattan, S.I.S. and Clark, B.F.C. Kinetin delays the onset of ageing characteristics in human fibroblasts. *Biochem Biophys Res* 1994;201:665-672.

11. Kowalska, E. Influence of kinetin (6-furfurylo-amino-purine) on human fibroblasts in the cell culture. *Folia Morphol* 1992;51:109-118.

12. Sharma, S.P., et al. Plant-growth hormone kinetin delays aging, prolongs the life-span and slows down development of the fruitfly Zaprionus paravittiger. *Biochem Biophys Res Comm* 1995;216:1067-1071.

13. Vicanova, J., et al. Epidermal and dermal characteristics in skin equivalent after systemic and topical application of skin care ingredients. *Ann N Y Acad Sci* 2006;1067:337-342.

14. Kimura, T. and Doi, K. Depigmentation and rejuvenation effects of kinetin on the aged skin of hairless descendants of Mexican hairless dogs. *Rejuvenation Res* 2004;7:32-39.

15. Hipkiss, A.R. On the "struggle between chemistry and biology during aging"—implications for DNA repair, apoptosis and proteolysis, and a novel route of intervention. *Biogerontology* 20012:173-178.

16. Orr, M.F. and McSwain, B. The effect of kinetin, kinetin ribofuranoside and gibberellic acid upon cultures of skin and mammary carcinoma and cystic disease. *Cancer Research* 1960;20:1362-1364.

17. Gallo, R.C., et al. Isopentenyladenosine stimulates and inhibits mitosis of human lymphocytes treated with phytohemagglutinin. *Science* 1969;165:400-402.

18. Mookerjee, B.K. et al. Effects of plant cytokinins on human lymphocyte transformation. *J Reticuloendothel Soc* 1979;25:299-314.

19. Saito, T., et al. Inhibitory effect of cytokinins on PHA-induced human lymphocyte stimulation. *Esperientia* 1979;35:685-686.

20. Adair, W.L. and Brennan, S.L. The role of N-6-isopentenyl adenine in tumor cell growth. *Biochem Biophys Res Commun* 1986;137:208-214.

21. Johnson, G.S., et al. N6-substituted adenines induce cell elongation irrespective of the intracellular cyclic AMP levels. *Exp Cell Res* 1974;85:47-56.

22. Dolezal, K, et al. Preparation and biological activity of 6-benzylaminopurine derivatives in plants and human cancer cells. *Bioorg Med Chem* 2006;14:875-874.

23. Ishii, Y. et al. Control of differentiation and apoptosis of human myeloid leukemia cells by cytokinins and cytokinin nucleosides, plant redifferentiation-inducing hormones. *Cell Growth Diff* 2002;13:19-26.

24. Ishii, Y, et al. Immediate up-regulation of the calcium-binding protein S100P and its involvement in the cytokinin-induced differentiation of human myeloid leukemia cells. *Biochim Biophys Acta* 2005;1745:156-165.

25. Berge, U., et al. Kinetin-induced differentiation of normal human keratinocytes undergoing aging in vitro. *Ann N Y Acad Sci* 2006;1067:332-336.

26. Vermeulen, K., et al. Antiproliferative effect of plant cytokinin analogues with an inhibitory activity on cyclin-dependent kinases. *Leukemia* 2002;16:299-305.

27. Dolezal, K., et al. Preparation and biological activity of 6-benzylaminopurine derivatives in plants and human cancer cells. *Bioorg Med Chem* 2006;14:875-884.

28. Olsen, A., et al. N(6)-Furfuryladenine, kinetin, protects against Fenton reaction-mediated oxidative damage to DNA. *Biochem Biophys Res Commun* 1999;256:499-502.

29. Hsiao, G., et al. Inhibitory activity of kinetin on free radical formation of activated platelets in vitro and on thrombus formation in vivo. *Eur J Pharm* 2003;465:281-287.

30. Sheu, J.R., et al. Inhibitory mechanisms of kinetin, a plant growth-promoting hormone, in platelet aggregation. *Platelets* 2003;14:189-196.

31. Kris-Etherton, P.M., et al. The effects of nuts on coronary heart disease risk. *Nutr Rev* 2001;59:103-111.

32. Hu, F.B., et al. Frequent nut consumption and risk of coronary heart disease in women: prospective cohort study. *BMJ* 1998;317:1341-1345.

33. Fraser, G.E., et al. A possible protective effect of nut consumption on risk of coronary heart disease. The Adventist Health Study. *Arch Intern Med* 1992;152:1416-1424.

34. Fife, B. *Coconut Cures: Preventing and Treating Common Health Problems with Coconut.* Colorado Springs, CO: Piccadilly Books. 2005.

35. Lindeberg, S. and Lundh, B. Apparent absence of stroke and ischaemic heart disease in a traditional Melanesian island: a clinical study in Kitava. *J Intern Med* 1993;233:269-275.
36. Dayrit, C.S. Coconut oil: atherogenic or not? *Philip J Cardiology* 2003;31:97-104.
37. Reed, M.J., et al. Acceleration of wound healing in aged rats by topical application of transforming growth factor-beta(1). *Wound Repair Regen* 1995;3:330-339.
38. Verallo-Rowell, V.M. *Rx: Coconuts! The Perfect Health Nut.* Xlibris. 2005.
39. Mamaril, J.C., et al. Enhancement of seedling growth with extracts from coconut water. *Philipp J Crop Sci* 1988;13:1-7.
40. Barciszewski, J., et al. Kinetin—a multiactive molecule. *International Journal of Biological Macromolecules* 2007;40:182-192.

Chapter 7: Gastrointestinal Health

1. Biffi, A., et al. Antiproliferative effect of fermented milk on the growth of a human breast cancer cell line. *Nutrition and Cancer* 1997;28:93-99.
2. Veer, P., et al. Consumption of fermented milk products and breast cancer: a case-control study in The Netherlands. *Cancer Res* 1989;49:4020-4023.

Chapter 8: Coconut Water Detox

1. Goldstein, J. *Triumph Over Disease by Fasting and Natural Diet.* New York: Arco Publishing Company. 1977.
2. Kano, M., et al. Changes in intestinal motility, visceral sensitivity and minor mucosal inflammation after fasting therapy in a patient with irritable bowel syndrome. *Journal of Gastroenterology and Hepatology* 2006;21:1078-1079.
3. Kanazawa, M. and Fukudo, S. Effects of fasting therapy on irritable bowel syndrome. *International Journal of Behavioral Medicine* 2006;13:214-220.
4. Michalsen, A., et al. Incorporation of fasting therapy in an integrative medicine ward: evaluation of outcome, safety, and effects on lifestyle adherence in a large prospective cohort study. *J Altern Complement Med* 2005;11:601-607.

5. Kjeldsen-Kragh, J, et al. Changes in laboratory variables in rheumatoid arthritis patients during a trial of fasting and one-year vegetarian diet. *Scand J Rheumatol* 1995;24:85-93.

6. Lithell, H, et al. A fasting and vegetarian diet treatment trial on chronic inflammatory disorders. *Acta Derm Venereol* 1983;63:397-403.

7. Kjeldsen-Kragh, J, et al. Controlled trial of fasting and one-year vegetarian diet in rheumatoid arthritis. *Lancet* 1991;338:899-902.

Index

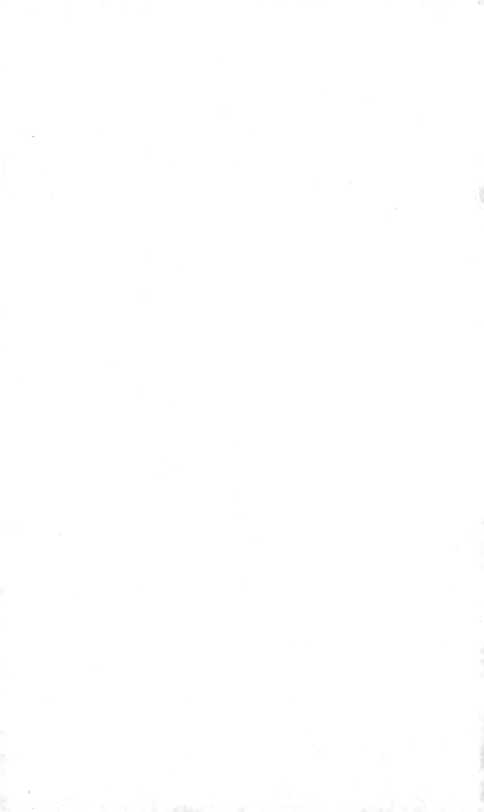